For my Father, to whom I bid my last farewell during this project:

Thanks for the continued support even to the conclusion of this work despite not having opportunity to see it for yourself. Thanks for believing in me through every unanticipated twist in life's bypaths. Thanks for being a dad, most especially my dad.

I love you always, even to the final end...

MUSIC UN-THERAPY HANDBOOK

THE ULTIMATE INTRODUCTORY GUIDE FOR USING SOUND DAILY TO ENHANCE WELLNESS AND EMBRACE QUALITY OF LIFE

D.L. SILVEY

CONTENTS

INTRODUCTION

In sound we are born, in sound we are healed.

— MEHTAB BENTON

Although we already intuitively understand that music makes us feel good, it has much more to offer. The concept of "music un-therapy," as I like to call it, embraces wellness and a quality of life that many people are largely unaware of. Scientific principles, such as anatomy and physiology, teach us that there are physical benefits from regular exercise routines; conceptually, these same principles can be applied using sound and music to benefit quality of life. We can take advantage of sonic resources daily to improve our physical, mental and emotional health and continue to learn more about their therapeutic properties as we implement them in clinical settings.

Research supports that using sound and music for medical applications has shown promise for various neurological and physical conditions, including Parkinson's disease, brain injuries, seizures, and the facilitation of the grieving, traumatic, depressive, and anxious processes in individuals. Music is something that virtually anyone can access. It can support treatment plans, medications, and therapy and help people reach a level of wellness synergistically that other healing modalities cannot attain by themselves. But as importantly, it is an easy energy source to incorporate, enhancing the vitality of your daily life.

Since the beginning of time, people have used music and sound to uplift, energize, calm, pacify, and even ease troubled spirits. It's no secret that a catchy, upbeat song can get our hearts racing and that a lovely melody can take us back to a pleasant memory or simply help us to relax. But there is a lot more to sound than we may recognize. Nature itself emits various sounds that are beyond our range of hearing. Even ferns and mushrooms produce music, which can be heard with the proper listening devices.

There are a variety of ways to use sound, which include cutting materials (yes, it is possible to cut with sound!), purifying water, stimulating rain, sonar, ultrasound imaging, ultrasonic cleaning, sonochemistry, lithotripsy (a noninvasive procedure that physically destroys hardened masses like kidney stones, bezoars, or gallstones), eliminating plastic pollution from water, and inspecting the integrity of machinery in factories and mechanic shops without having to open the equipment. It is also used by therapists, healers, and medical professionals to strengthen and treat the body and mind. In an alternative setting, modern energy healers also employ a variety of frequencies, binaural beats, and other sound modalities to effect spectacular wellness results.

I've worked as an X-ray technologist for over ten years and have seventeen years of prior public speaking and interpersonal communication experience. However, through my involvement as a keyboardist, composer, and sound designer, I've grown to become a sound and music enthusiast at heart. My interactions with sound and music have led me to realize that they are sources of abundant healing that are much more easily accessible, produced, and used than most traditional forms of therapy. I want to share what I've learned through music and sound with anyone open to change and transformation so they can live healthier, happier, and more self-actualized lives.

Most of us have easy access to many advantages recognized by the field of music therapy. This little-known but incredibly effective therapeutic technique can be applied to many situations. It involves a lot more than just playing your favorite song. It targets a particular problem by using sound and music to engage the brain in specific ways. Although the full experience typically requires a board-certified practitioner, you can still apply several of the methodologies in your regular, daily life. Suppose you are considering consulting a music therapist. In that case, this book will introduce you to some of the basic principles of music therapy that can be implemented outside the clinical setting while also demonstrating how to put them into practice in your own life.

Un-therapy differs from conventional psychology because it doesn't prioritize mending past wounds. The people who can use this mental technology are not considered patients because they do not have emotional or psychological disorders and are not labeled as "ill." Instead, they are regarded as clients of un-therapy. The foundation of un-therapy is the concept that we can control only two things: our thoughts and behavior. People are taught how to reflect on and change the attitudes and behaviors that keep them in unfavorable circumstances. Combining music therapy and un-therapy offers us a revolutionary and progressive methodology that we can use to manage our moods, calm our racing thoughts, and heal our minds and bodies on a regular basis. All it takes is incorporating a few simple music therapy concepts into our daily routine.

There are numerous other applications for sound. Scientists are beginning to understand multiple ways in which sound can positively impact mood, brain function, and healing. Anyone with a cell phone, a musical instrument of any kind, a bowl and a stick, or actually nothing more than their lips and voice to hum and sing with can access sound healing for free. For a deeper understanding of the healing effects of sound and music, let's embark on a journey through the fascinating world of music un-therapy.

1

MUSIC, SOUND, AND THERAPY THROUGH THE AGES

The power of music to integrate and cure... is quite fundamental. It is the profoundest non-chemical medication.

— OLIVER SACKS

SOUND THROUGH THE AGES

From horns honking in the street to the pings on your cell phone, today's world can seem like a very noisy place. But things weren't always like this. There weren't always ambient sounds traveling through the air, and there weren't always people and animals nearby to produce these environmental sounds. Indeed, there haven't always been sound recording technologies available, now prevalent virtually everywhere, whether in subway cars, posh studios, or basements. From the very first sound that was ever produced to the first sound that an animal heard or the first sound that a human being recorded, sound has a history. Over time, as this world has evolved, numerous discoveries and advancements have contributed to the vast realm of sound and music that we now experience.

Ancient Philosophers and Scientists

Before the realization that sound travels in waves, many people were perplexed and interested in how we could hear what we heard. Everything changed when some of the most eminent scientists of early eras discovered how sound travels.

Aristotle, a Greek philosopher, was one of the first to assert that sound travels in waves. According to Aristotle, sound waves propagate as far as possible while maintaining their sonic properties.

The first individual to document the connection between a wave's frequency and the respective pitch it generates was Italian physicist Galileo. Galileo was able to draw this conclusion by observing the results of using a chisel to scrape against a brass plate. Furthermore, he noted that the spacing between the grooves — produced due to the chisel's contact with the brass plate — varied in direct proportion to the resulting screech's pitch. This vital discovery helped to define why the pitch and character of the sound waves produced by musical instruments vary.

After discovering that sound is propagated by waves, people became curious about the speed at which these waves moved.

In 1640, French mathematician Marin Mersenne became the first to document the speed of sound as it moved through the atmosphere. As science and technology advanced, it was determined that Mersenne's speed of sound was off by less than ten percent. Even though ten percent may seem like a significant error for such data, his findings are quite remarkable given the primitive state of technology during his time.

Twenty years after Mersenne's findings, a British scientist named Robert Boyle concluded that sound must pass through a medium in order to propagate or transfer. The molecular composition of the air itself serves as this medium. Boyle conducted an experiment in which he put a ringing bell inside a glass jar and extracted the air. From the results, he was able to draw his conclusion. He observed that the noise of the bell's ringing diminished until it could not be heard as the air was evacuated from the jar. The absence of air prevented any sound from being transmitted, so no sound stimulus was present to reach his ears.

Shamanic Healers and Spiritualists

Sound and music are potent cures. The history of using music and sound for healing is extensive and diverse.

Ancient civilizations used sound as one of the numerous therapeutic methods to treat a wide range of illnesses long before the development of contemporary medical technology and medications. For instance, around 4000 BC, high priests in ancient Egypt used the seven vowel sounds in their rituals to uplift the spirit and speed up healing processes.

Around 500 BC, Pythagoras, attributed as the original inventor of music therapy, established the Pythagoras Mystery School on the island of Crotona to promote the use of the flute and lyre as the primary instruments for healing. He also created the mono-chord, a single-stringed musical instrument with the tension provided by a fixed weight. It opened the door for Pythagoras to decipher the enigmas of musical intervals and learn that healing could occur using sound and harmonic frequencies that were performed to what he called "soul adjustments."

The Aborigines, the oldest known cultural group in Australia, are thought to have used the didgeridoo, also known as yidaki, for 40,000 years to accelerate the healing of wounds, illnesses, and various types of broken bones. The didgeridoo emits sounds that are interestingly compatible with contemporary sound healing technology.

American armed forces also used sound therapy in 1945 to aid in recovering World War II combatants. Many people refer to this as the official start of implementing the practice of music therapy as a viable medical resource.

20th-Century Scientists

Through the 1700s and 1800s, scientists continued to study waves in general and sound waves in particular. Due to techno-logical advancements and knowledge gained from early experi-ments and minor discoveries, numerous scientists and mathematicians started researching the subject in depth. One of them was the French mathematician Joseph Fourier, who observed that a vibrating string produces a series of waves that move periodically.

Arguably, the most significant discovery related to sound waves is attributed to Austrian physicist Christian Doppler, who created mathematical formulae defining the frequency of sound waves based on the relative motion of the wave source and observer. Doppler also concluded that the medium in which sound waves travel affects their velocity. In a simplified context, according to his theory, sound intensity decreases as the wave source moves farther away from an observer because the waves' frequency drops. On the other hand, if the wave source moves closer to the observer, the sound becomes louder and more intense. This phenomenon is known as the Doppler effect.

You can think of it in this respect; consider how an emergency vehicle's sound changes when standing on the street. As it approaches, the sirens get louder. After the vehicle passes you, the sound softens and drops in pitch. This same principle can be applied medically using ultrasound to determine blood flow properties or locate strictures in veins and arteries.

More specifically relevant to music, in the late 1890s, Harvard physicist Wallace Sabine made a significant discovery regarding music performance. Prior to Sabine's discovery, very little attention was given to the acoustic space in which musicians performed. Sabine was tasked with enhancing the acoustics of a Harvard Museum, leading him to take reverberation measurements and experiment with materials that absorb sound. He realized that even a venue's seating plays a role in its acoustic character. His work ultimately led to the development of scientifically designed concert halls, such as the Boston Symphony Hall, which opened in 1900. Today, all concert halls are built with careful consideration for the acoustic character, a development made possible by Sabine's work.

USE OF SOUND TODAY

Today's world is inconceivable without sound. It is the first sensation we have when we wake up in the morning and the last sense we experience before going to sleep at night. Every day, we immerse ourselves in the world around us through sound by engaging in conversations, listening to music, watching television, listening to podcasts, and engaging in any variety of other activities that we take for granted.

No matter the source, sound always functions in a similar fashion: It is the energy created when something vibrates. We frequently consider only the psychological aspect of sound, which is the process by which those vibrations are transformed into something we perceive as words, music, and other noises in our ears to be interpreted by our brains. But sound is more than just an intangible idea; it also has physical components, and the waves that constitute sound have been used in a plethora of fascinating applications.

Sound can be implemented to do more than simply entertain us on our way to work or to 'while away' an afternoon because sound is an actual, physical wave. Thus, regulated sound is also employed in treating illnesses, cleaning, producing electricity, and creating one-of-a-kind works of art. The uses for sound listed below are just a few among a myriad of sonic benefits that many of us may be unaware of.

Sonar Technology

Sound navigation and ranging, or sonar, is used to explore and map large bodies of water and their underlying terrain because sound waves travel farther in water than radar and light waves. It is additionally used to detect objects' location — as fish or other vessels — in the ocean utilizing acoustic sound waves. The most straightforward sonar systems employ a transducer to emit a sound pulse and then carefully monitor the time it takes for the sound pulse to return to the transducer.

During World War I, sonar was created to locate icebergs and submarines. During World War II, significant advancements in this technology were made. Eventually, scientists modified the extremely sensitive apparatus for use in oceanographic research. The more sophisticated the sonar system, the more direction and range information it can provide. It is possible to estimate an object's distance using this time difference and the speed of sound in water (roughly 1,500 meters per second).

Water Purification

Due to a lack of water resources and the harm caused by sewage treatment processes for aquatic life, water filtration has become more and more crucial. The cutting-edge technology developed for purifying water takes advantage of the properties of ultrasonic waves. This technology functions as a more sophisticated form of oxidation, aiding in the removal of various contaminants. The fundamental idea behind ultrasound is the destruction of bacterial cells and organic materials that are hard to break down through other means.

Membrane filtration, a term used to describe a variety of procedures using synthetic membranes to isolate chemicals and other substances, is now recognized as the primary technology for separating pollutants from contaminated water sources and thereby implemented for water purification. To meet the ever-stricter requirements for drinking water and uphold public confidence, membrane processes are a critical component of conventional water treatment systems.

The idea of employing ultrasound during membrane filtration is primarily based on the ultrasound cavitation effect. Like all sound waves, ultrasound travels through a series of molecule-driven compression and decompression waves. Ceramic filters can be cleaned quickly and affordably using ultrasound-generated bubbles in the water. When the bubbles pop, their energy is released as tiny but ferociously strong jets of water that clean the filter's surface and flush out debris.

Music Therapy

Music therapy is used in medical applications to help reduce stress, boost moods, and encourage self-expression. It is a well-respected form of treatment in the medical field, with a plethora of research and results to support it. Experiences with music therapy may involve listening, singing, playing an instrument, or writing music. Despite preconceived notions, it is not a prerequisite to have well developed musical aptitudes or skills to participate.

In 1945, the US War Department developed and applied formal music therapy for the first time. It offered military service members recovering in Army hospitals occupational therapy, education, entertaining activities, and physical conditioning. The patient and therapist would engage in one or more of the following activities during music therapy:

- **Create:** Make music by writing lyrics and/or music or by working collaboratively.
- **Sing:** Vocal expression of their music or the works of others.
- **Listen:** Appreciate and/or analyze music and lyrics.
- **Move:** Ranging from as simple as tapping their toes to music or as elaborate as dancing a routine or even freestyle.
- **Explore lyrics:** Discuss the meaning of a song's lyrics along with evaluating the emotions and memories they invoke.
- **Play an instrument:** Actively engaging in the music by playing the piano, guitar, drums, etc.

It should be noted for you as the reader that you are encouraged to implement these very resources to enhance your own quality of life and support ongoing wellness especially in the absence of any illness or malady. This is the core essence and intent of these writings; to exercise and benefit *daily* from such noted activities that have and are proving themselves effective within institutional settings. Include partnering with friends, family, neighbors or co-workers where you can mutually benefit each other with these interactive sessions and activities.

Medical Application

While ultrasound waves can't be heard, they are used daily to diagnose and treat patients. In the past 40 years, ultrasound imaging has advanced from creating blurry, monochromatic images to producing crisp, three-dimensional images in real-time. New technologies are constantly being developed.

When used for medical diagnostics, ultrasound typically ranges in frequency from 1 to 15 megahertz (MHz), is directed at a target, and is received by a transducer. The signal is next translated into visual information, signal curves, or audible sounds.

Three broad categories can be used to classify the use of medical ultrasound:

1. imaging for diagnosis
2. medium-power therapeutic applications for purposes like muscle warming and stimulation
3. high-powered therapeutic applications, including dissolving kidney stones and treating neurological conditions like essential tremors

In diagnostic procedures called echocardiography, ultrasound was first used to examine the heart. This technology's implementations are as diverse as cranial studies, monitoring fetus development during pregnancy, evaluating tumors and other lesions along with providing support for many medical processes. Ultrasound can be used to analyze any tissue, organ, joint, or large vein or artery in the body.

For instance, ultrasound imaging employs the doppler effect to gauge blood flow in an artery. The frequency of the reflected wave will change with the speed of the reflector, much like the previously mentioned analogy of an ambulance passing by your house. In other words, if a blood cell is moving toward you, the frequency will be higher; if it is moving away from you, the frequency will be lower.

Ultrasound is regarded as the safest method for examining the function of internal organs. Sound waves are induced into the body. The sound waves which are reflected back are used to produce images of the heart, liver, veins, and other body structures. Additionally, the heart's beat and blood flow rate can be measured. Other techniques, such as CT or MRI scans, aren't as effective for dynamic flow evaluation.

SOUND AS A WAY OF LIFE

Every aspect of our lives is impacted by sound, including how we communicate. Although ears pick up sounds from the environment, the brain interprets and comprehends these sounds. Our capacity to hear and sense vibration is essential for giving us knowledge about the world around us.

The brain's auditory cortex, which is found in the temporal lobe, is uniquely equipped to process and make sense of the sounds we hear. It enables humans to interpret speech and other environmental sounds.

The Power of Words

Words are powerful. They have the capacity to both create and destroy. Words have energy and power. They can uplift, heal, interfere, restrict, hurt, and humble. Sometimes, merely one word can make all the difference; words are among humanity's most potent forces at its disposal. We can use this force destructively by speaking words of despair or constructively by speaking words of encouragement.

Positive words, like "peace" and "love," can influence how genes are expressed, promoting the development of certain frontal lobe regions and improving cognitive function. They activate the brain's motivational centers and strengthen resiliency.

On the other hand, hostile language can sabotage particular genes crucial for producing stress-relieving neurochemicals. This triggers anxiety, where most of our thought processes default, because it is ingrained in human nature as a way for our primal brain instincts to protect us from threats promoting survival. But in the end, it only causes us harm.

The activity in our amygdala, the brain's fear center, can be triggered by solely one unfavorable word. As a result, many stress-inducing hormones and neurotransmitters are released, impairing more rational brain functions; this is particularly true of logic, reason, and language. Angry words trigger alarm signals in the brain which partially shut down the frontal lobe's centers for logic and reasoning.

Some of us have the bad habit of reiterating redundant derogatory phrases. The issue is that a word or phrase's influence over us grows as we use it more frequently. Interestingly, it makes no difference whether the information is accurate or not. The frequency of exposure is the only factor that has an impact.

Words, spoken or heard, carry emotional power. Every phrase we choose to elicit can have a profound effect. A manager's, mentor's, or boss's words might initially seem unimportant. However, the significance of words should never be underestimated; regard every one of them instead as impactful. Words have the power to uplift or demoralize, they can inspire or dishearten. Relationships and personal interactions at work and in our social circles are forged through words. Relationships are strengthened or strained by them. Simply put, language has the immense, colossal power to bring about change — whether for the better or worse.

The Influence of Music

Music is a deeply personal experience for everyone. It has the power to affect mood, perception, and change. From generation to generation, music has shaped cultures and societies all over the world.

The human experience has always been infused with music, from the drumbeats of our prehistoric ancestors to the limitless streaming services of today. Our emotional states and moods can be profoundly influenced by music. When we need motivation and inspiration, music provides it for us. It can comfort us when we are anxious, lift our spirits when we are down, and inspire us again when we are discouraged. We form connections with people through music, especially those who compose or perform it; we sing along to their lyrics, dance to their beats, and identify with them because of their offering through self-expression.

Studies have demonstrated that listening to music can boost happiness and reduce anxiety. Recent studies have found that even sad music can be comforting. However, as the product of our combined individual experiences, we already know this intuitively. How frequently has your mood changed when your favorite tune began to play, and how often have you felt relaxed having music keep you company during a long commute?

Researchers have speculated about music's potential therapeutic and mood-enhancing effects for centuries. Over time, regular exposure to energetic and joyful music helps to elevate moods and increase happiness. And happiness is almost universally correlated with improved physical health, increased income, and stimulating relationships.

When dealing with a profound interpersonal loss, such as the end of a cherished relationship, sad music can be especially uplifting and soothing. It often serves as a validation of what someone might be experiencing. It can be compared to spending time with a friend who deeply understands your situation.

Medical professionals are more and more employing music therapy programs to assist patients with a range of conditions, including pain relief, memory enhancement, and stress management. According to extensive research, patients who listened to music before, during, or after surgery felt less pain and anxiety than those who did not. Singing lyrics can be constructive for people whose left side of the brain, which governs speech, has been damaged by a stroke or other form of brain trauma. Because singing comes from the right side of the brain, which is unharmed in this case, people can learn to speak their thoughts by beginning with a melody then progressively over time, can ultimately stop having to do so.

When you listen to music or play an instrument, the memory, reasoning, speech, emotion, and reward-related brain regions are all activated. Not only does music aid in reminiscing previously held memories, but it also aids in creating fresh ones. Songs and melodies have the potential to shape people's identities, motivate them, and direct their behavior. Music can unite people, ignite the imagination, and encourage creativity even when enjoyed in solitude. Music is often a prominent factor for the many people attempting to connect with others and determine their place in their community. But the inverse can be equally true, that one who has genuinely been influenced by music is never alone.

Music is a potent force able to unite societies by giving the voiceless a platform, influencing moods and promoting inspiration, encouraging us to move and dance, and bridging communication gaps by fostering knowledge and idea exchange.

EXERCISE

Think for a moment about all the ways music influences your life. This is often something we like to explore about ourselves. Make a list of the occasions surrounding your life when you typically decide to listen to music. Why those specific instances? What kind of music is your go-to for these occasions? Do you have specific playlists for them?

How does music contribute to those moments? Consider how you feel when you listen to music in these situations, whether while working from home, traveling, attending a party, spending time with friends and family, or simply relaxing alone.

We do well to take the time to consider the immense scope of sound and music, not just in terms of genres and styles but also in terms of technicalities, applications, and influences. By understanding the science behind it, we can strive to explore and understand how beneficial sound can be to our everyday lives.

2

SOUND SCIENCE

THE FUNDAMENTALS OF SOUND

Sound is a form of energy created by vibrations. On a technical note, these vibrations produced by objects in motion cause the molecules of the atmosphere around it to respond at the same frequency as the dominant vibration. These molecules, in turn, collide with additional molecules, causing them to vibrate as well. This molecular chain reaction persists until the original energy level is expended through the various collisions; this chain of events represents what is known as a sound wave. Despite the numerous molecular collisions as the sound wave travels through the air, the air molecules are not displaced; each molecule moves away from a stationary point when disturbed but eventually returns to its original position. These concepts of molecular interactions also apply to the cells and molecules in your brain and body, which in part, become the stimuli for producing and interpreting sound.

When we hear something, we are actually sensing air vibrations. The vibrations that enter the outer ear cause our eardrums to vibrate or oscillate. Three tiny bones, the malleus (hammer), the incus (anvil), and the stapes (stirrup), are affixed to the eardrum, so they vibrate as well. These middle ear bones strengthen incoming vibrations, amplifying them before the auditory nerve is exposed to the vibrational stimuli relaying the signal to the appropriate brain region for interpretation.

The properties of sound are altered as they pass through various media consisting of gas, liquid, or solid matter. A wave moves more quickly through a medium with higher density than it would through one of lower density. In other words, sound travels more quickly through water than air and faster through bone than water.

When a medium vibrates, its molecules may move vertically or horizontally. The sound energy that causes the molecules to move back and forth, or oscillate, in the direction of the sound's motion is referred to as a longitudinal wave. The up-and-down molecular vibration produces transverse waves, which occur perpendicular to the wave's direction of propagation.

In a more practical sense, every sound we hear in our everyday environment consists of combinations of simple sounds. Speaking and hearing both involve complex interactions of these vibrations. Air passes through our vocal cords when we speak, causing them to vibrate. We alter the sounds produced by varying the amount of tension exerted on the vocal cords.

Vocal cords can be extended to raise their tonal quality or loosened to produce lower sounds. This higher/lower tone relationship is known as the sound's pitch.

Tone describes a musical sound's characteristics. When a tuning fork is struck, a single frequency of sound, known as a pure tone, is produced. However, when we sing or play a note on a trumpet or violin, we combine a fundamental frequency with additional frequencies (known as harmonics or overtones) to produce very distinct, unique sounds. This imparts a definitive sound for each musical instrument.

As with other waves, sound waves have physical properties such as wavelength, frequency, and amplitude. As opposed to different types of waves, for example, surface ocean waves, these characteristics are not as readily visible or apparent. Fortunately, the eardrum, or tympanic membrane, which divides the inner ear from the outer ear, enables us to distinguish these traits. The pitch of a sound wave (the high or low sound characteristic) is defined by its wavelength and frequency. A tuba, for instance, is a low-frequency instrument and thus produces a low pitch. The volume of a sound wave is denoted by its amplitude.

SOUND IN NATURE

Interestingly, plants use a variety of means to interact with their surroundings, including chemical secretions, chemical shapes, and colors; additionally, plants communicate through sound. As humans, we are familiar with the sound of the wind rustling through the trees or the sound of leaves and pine needles as they sway. However, each species possesses its own unique sonic signature; conifers have a different rustling sound distinguishable from maples. This is comparable to the variations in human vocal tones produced by the vocal cords' physiological resonance frequency. Regarding vegetation, each tree and plant species has a distinctive sound based on a morphological expression.

However, the bioacoustics of plants goes far beyond these transient sounds that are audible to humans. Evidence indicates plants produce audible, infrasonic, and ultrasonic acoustic emissions. The belief is that physiological vascular processes produce plant acoustic emissions as a byproduct. Air bubbles in the xylem system were once thought to cause such acoustic emissions from trees; however, more recent evidence now suggests that plants produce sound emissions independent of cavitation disruptions.

Various plants' germination, growth, and behavioral responses to sound have been well documented, as have measured sound emissions from diverse vegetation. Sound waves are efficiently conducted through the soil and require little energy to generate. Consequently, plants interpret their environment and surroundings using sound. According to preliminary research, sound is produced in the root tips when a plant's cell wall breaks. A plant's root will only react to sound waves that match the frequencies that the plant itself emits. This may imply that as a form of underground communication, plants can recognize and translate sonic vibrations into signals that cause behavioral changes.

Plants emit audio acoustic emissions (AAE) between 10 and 240 hertz (Hz) and ultrasonic acoustic emissions (UAE) between 20 and 300 kilohertz (kHz). Among these diverse botanical mechanisms, sound vibrations may be a key component. When roots are exposed to unidirectional 220 Hz sound stimuli, they grow toward the vibration's source. This supports the theory that plants can convert mechanical triggers into neural signals. Electrograph vibrational detection has been used to capture loud, frequent clicks along the elongation zone of corn plant root tips. These are recognized as emissions of structured sound waves. Even when cut off from contact with neighboring plants affecting the subsequent exchange of chemical and light signals, plants can still sense their neighbors and locate relatives. Additionally, various plants have been found to emit UAE, believed to be caused by collapsing water columns under intense strain.

The Audible Spectrum

The characteristics of human hearing differ from the hearing of other animals. The auditory field is perceived by our ears as a specific frequency and intensity range, meaning we can hear sounds within a particular range of pitches and volumes. Other animals, however, can sense acoustic vibrations outside of this domain.

Humans and animals hear by detecting vibrations transmitted as sound waves in the air, ground, or water. These vibrations are captured within the middle ear and converted into pressure waves, which are then conducted to the inner ear or cochlea - a fluid-filled structure designed to translate sound. The cochlea transforms these waves into signals that can be interpreted by the auditory brain region.

In addition to volume, a sound's low and high pitch determines the range of human hearing. Volume is measured in decibels (dB), while pitch is measured in hertz (Hz). Infrasound refers to sounds below the human audible range, and ultrasound is a term used to describe sounds higher than the perceptible range.

For someone with normal, healthy hearing, the human audible pitch range begins at around 20 Hz, comparable to the lowest pedal on a pipe organ. The upper extreme for human hearing is 20,000 Hz, which is the highest frequency that can audibly be experienced without discomfort. The auditory range, however, is most sensitive between 2,000 and 5,000 Hz.

Despite having a relatively broad hearing range, humans cannot hear certain sounds, take for example a dog whistle, because these sounds fall outside the human audible range. Dogs, on the contrary, have no difficulty hearing the device because they have a much broader range of hearing than we do at higher frequencies. Additionally, lower-frequency sounds, such as the roar of a wind turbine, are frequently felt as vibrations rather than heard as sounds to humans because these fall below our range of hearing.

Bridging the Gap

Despite being unable to hear many sounds produced in and by nature because of their being outside the human audible range, curious individuals have made it possible to listen to the bioacoustics of plants!

Although it has been a practice since the 1920s, bioacoustics only officially became a field of study in the 1960s. Large microphones and sound equipment were carried by ecologists as they moved about, recording wildlife sounds and manually tallying the species they saw. Some had to trek through forests using car batteries to power their recording equipment. It took a lot of time and resources to review the acoustic data manually following carrying their cumbersome equipment through diverse countryside and walking for extended periods. The introduction and evolving power of machine learning and the development of smaller, less expensive, and automatic recording devices have given the field of bioacoustics new life and energy, ushering in a new era of acoustic conservation. Machine-learning algorithms can be trained to recognize target animal calls and human activity like logging while analyzing the health of ecosystems and tropical forests instead of researchers manually listening to thousands of hours of acoustic data.

In the late 1970s, in Italy's internationally famous cultural region of Damanhur, a device that can convert the electromagnetic impulse of plants into melodies was created. Oberto Airaudi (also known as Falco Tarassaco), the creator of Damanhur, and his associates spent significant time researching the bioelectric processes that occur in plants, trees, and flowers. During their investigation, they created a tool to detect electromagnetic variations from a plant's leafy surface to its roots and translate them into sound. They found that conductivity is a crucial sign of a plant's vitality, generating important channels for water, minerals, and other nutrients inside trees and flowers.

The idea that plants have different innate intelligence and logic from humans is being supported more and more by science. We are becoming more aware of nature's innate ability to speak to us when we have the means to listen. This awareness has led to extensive research that still persists today.

Experimental Discovery

A microphone was placed 10 cm from select plants by Itzhak Khait and his colleagues at Tel Aviv University in Israel. It picked up sounds in the ultrasonic range of 20 to 100 kHz (Vaughan, 2019). Through this experiment, they discovered that when tomato and tobacco plants were stressed due to a lack of water or when their stem was cut, they produced sounds outside the range of human hearing. However, even up to 5 m away, insects and some mammals could hear and react to these sounds. It has even been suggested that plants may be able to hear when other plants are dehydrated and respond accordingly. Researchers hypothesize that a moth might decide not to lay eggs on a plant that sounds water-stressed.

It has been noted that different stress levels trigger a variance in the plant sounds emitted. By instructing a machine learning model to distinguish between the sounds of the plants and the wind, rain, and other noises in a greenhouse, researchers were able to reliably determine, in most cases, whether the stress was brought on by dryness or by a cut, based on the sound's intensity and frequency. For instance, cut tobacco makes more intense noises than water-hungry tobacco. These discoveries may change the way we perceive the plant kingdom, which up until now, was perceived to be largely silent.

PlantWave

One of today's most popular tools for enjoying the sounds of nature is the PlantWave device. This device can serve as a bridge between people and nature through its sonic interpretations. It employs a characteristic algorithm that has undergone extensive research to convert electrical signals into sound. Every organism has a different pulse stream, and every plant has a distinctive biological signature sound.

The team developed the software algorithm to transform plant behavior into audible signals for improved communication that humans can understand. Two electrodes link the device to the plant; one is placed on a leaf, and the other is inserted into the soil near the plant's roots. Through this methodology, a sonic window into the secret life of plants has been devised.

The researchers behind PlantWave have found that plants demonstrate it is possible for them to learn to communicate with people. The plants initially understand that the sounds produced by the instrument result from their electrical activity before learning to modulate it to alter the sounds. Over time, more advanced plants learn to modulate the sounds so as to communicate with people in a tangible way. They frequently communicate with musicians reiterating identical scales, tunes, and notes.

The PlantWave provides the option for the user to choose from various musical instruments, scales, root notes, and other options. The melody's original composer, however, is always the plant. Each plant is unique, as is each leaf on a plant itself. Their music is affected by outside factors like touch, moisture, movement, etc. Whenever a spike appears on the device, the notes change, presumably to the plant's preference. A plant that is underwatered might only play a few notes. In contrast, an exceptionally healthy and flourishing plant may play the entire range of notes. Sometimes a plant's response increases independently, possibly due to an interaction with an individual's presence, thoughts, or emotions.

THINGS WE CAN DISCOVER FROM SOUNDS WE CANNOT HEAR

This heading may seem an oxymoron since, theoretically, a "sound that cannot be heard" can hardly be classified as a sound. However, similar to how the tools, as mentioned earlier, pick up the plant music outside of our audible spectrum and give us insights into the secret life of plants, many other sounds that we cannot hear can be accessed through scientific instruments that can detect them and provide us with a wealth of helpful information.

Potential eruptions

Small earthquakes frequently occur before volcanic eruptions. When they do so in quick succession, they produce what is known as a harmonic tremor, which is a sustained release of infrasonic sound brought on by the movement of magma under extreme pressure. The Fuego Volcano in Guatemala, Arenal Volcano in Costa Rica, and Redoubt Volcano in Alaska are a few examples of volcanoes scientists have found to have produced these harmonic tremors before erupting.

An electret condenser microphone, developed to cancel out background noise, allows scientists to record and analyze this sonic phenomenon. These microphones are arranged underground in an array to capture the infrasonic emissions from the volcano. These signal emissions are then transmitted for processing through underground cables. These details, along with the seismic data from the volcano, can aid researchers in better understanding the activity that takes place inside a volcano just before an eruption.

Storm Location

When a hurricane passes through a region, it generates ocean waves interacting with other wave systems. These interactions between waves create a type of infrasound called a microbarom, which some people refer to as the voice of the sea. Microbaroms emit a limited range of low-frequency sounds that can be heard thousands of miles away, either as distinct energy bursts or as an ongoing oscillation. Though some of the frequencies are in the audibly range, most of the sound energy falls below the threshold of human hearing.

The National Center for Physical Acoustics is developing a mobile monitoring system to record these microbaroms. This system can be used to monitor a storm from several different locations. By analyzing the data gathered from the system, scientists can use triangulation to pinpoint the precise location of the storm, identify and gauge nearby wave conditions, and potentially save lives.

Nuclear Tests

Nuclear explosions occurring in the atmosphere or shallow underground can produce infrasonic waves that an infrasound network is designed to detect and identify. As a result, infrasound technology can assist in detecting illicit nuclear activity and detonation research in a region. It can collaborate with seismic technologies to identify and assess potential atmospheric and underground testing hazards.

The Preparatory Commission for the Comprehensive Nuclear-Test-Ban Treaty Organization (CTBTO) started setting up infrasound stations in 2001 in an effort to uncover covert nuclear testing by measuring the low-frequency sound waves that nuclear weapons disperse over long distances. The CTBTO's International Monitoring System (IMS) set up stations that record infrasound using microbarometers, sensitive devices calibrated to quickly measure variations in atmospheric pressure (Kiniry, 2013). These low-frequency sound waves are converted to electrical impulses by the microbarometer at the infrasound station before being transmitted via radio waves or fiber optics to a central recording facility. The signals are analyzed and processed by computers, which then prepare their findings for data transmission. This information is then transferred via satellite to a central facility in Vienna, where their origins are identified. With the aid of infrasound technology, the IMS was able to locate and determine the size of North Korea's first successful nuclear test in 2009.

Avalanche Detection

Even avalanches emit infrasound. Avalanches can be recognized using automated monitoring systems from safe locations far away from the active region where they occur. Scientists prefer using multiple-sensor monitoring systems to help pinpoint the locations of avalanches because wind noise can occasionally lead to incorrect readings in single-sensor monitoring systems. Avalanche-prone areas can become safer as a result. Even in the event that an unexpected avalanche occurs, the monitoring system can send automated alerts to assist locating those who might be trapped in the snow-flow more efficiently and quickly.

Elephant Behavior

Elephants communicate with one another using infrasound, just like many other animals, such as whales, pigeons, and hippos. Researchers have been examining this low-frequency communication to learn more about the mating behaviors of elephants and how these pachyderms can coordinate their movements when traveling in separate groups.

Elephant expert William Langbauer conducted an infrasound field study in Africa using a specially designed Pachyderm 2 loudspeaker that generates sounds below 60 Hz and records them at various ranges up to 125 yards away. He learned from this research that infrasound waves can pass unimpeded through air, leaves, and trees, all of which readily absorb higher-frequency sound waves. In doing so, he demonstrated infrasound as an ideal medium for long-distance communication. In fact, Langbauer calculates that elephants can hear infrasonic calls from a distance of more than 2-1/2 miles.

Bird Communication

Along the lines of animals incorporating infrasound in their endeavors for survival, according to Jonathan Hagstrum of the U.S. Geological Survey, birds use infrasound comparable to how people use GPS, by listening to low-frequency sound waves produced by the earth and using their origins as a guide to return home.

Pigeons and seabirds, in particular, are especially infrasound sensitive. Deep ocean waves are constantly generating acoustic energy. And that acoustic energy is transmitted through the earth as seismic energy before being reflected off the landscape and released once more into the atmosphere. Pigeons, seabirds, and other infrasound-sensitive birds are thought to listen to that reradiated infrasound and use this acoustic map to navigate to their homes.

CYMATICS: SOUND AS A VISUAL

Cymatics is a study of the visualization of audio frequency. The influence of sound on us is invisible, but it guides and shapes us. Waveforms can be visibly depicted when recording sound digitally. That, however, only provides a two-dimensional representation. However, the world of cymatics offers us a different perspective. It contributes significantly to our understanding of how sound affects each of us. According to cymatics, everything that we consider solid, including our bodies, is constantly vibrating at its own rate. This study demonstrates how sound, geometry, light, and mathematics are clearly merged into one by presenting stunning images made by frequencies of various sources present in our bodies, in nature, and beyond.

German physicist Ernst Chladni is renowned for generating simple geometric shapes by placing sand on a sonically controlled oscillating metal plate to study the physics of sound. Over a century later, Dr. Hans Jenny started experimenting with various liquids, solids, and continuously vibrating frequencies to further investigate the physics of sound. Using the Greek word Kyma, which means wave, he coined the term "cymatics." (Arnold, 2014)

The CymaScope

John Stuart Reid and Erik Larson created the CymaScope. This tool provides even more specific information about this developing research. Ultrapure water is given a sonic imprint, and digital cameras are used to capture the patterns created.

The Zero Point

Zero points generated by tones are manifest as patterns in water or on vibrating plates with sand or other substances. These nodes, or zero points, are regions devoid of vibration where the materials combine to create a visible pattern. It is incredible to discover that a tone does not impose a vibration across an entire surface but instead produces a variety of distinct, stunning geometric shapes, each with a unique pattern similar to snowflakes.

The image is slightly different in experiments using liquids. A tone causes a standing wave to form with timed peaks and valleys. The nodes or regions of lower vibration are represented by the troughs, while the harmonic content lifting the water is represented by the image's peaks.

These distinct and understated tones produce extraordinarily complex and beautiful cymatic images, which represent a peculiar type of geometry with recurring patterns like spheres, hexagons, and spirals. These natural components support revitalizing effects similar to lounging by the ocean or hiking in the woods. Conversely, imagine the effects that a combination of harsh or unnatural sounds have on our bodies if just one tone is able to leave these profound impressions. As we become more in tune with the natural world, we will undoubtedly become more conscious of what is healthful and adds substance to life and what the effects of urban noise pollution can do to unsettle it.

Although the study of cymatics initially focused on visual experiments, it has since expanded to cover metaphysical, philosophical, and environmental impact issues as well. The theory maintains that while increasing electromagnetic fields and noise pollution can throw us off balance or, in the worst-case scenario, cause blatant illness, the vibrational geometry of nature can restore our equilibrium. When we begin to consider the fundamental nature of vibration, everything becomes interconnected.

These varied aspects of sound reflect the complexity of sound itself. The energy that makes up these various sonic elements is intricate and abundant. It opens whole worlds of possibilities that we can access from exploring sound alone.

3

SOUND AS ENERGY

Physical sound can lead you to the inner vibration of Prana. Prana is the cause of all sound, and sound is the expression of Prana.

— SWAMI SATCHIDANANDA

WHAT IS SOUND ENERGY?

It is difficult to find a place in this world where noise is not a prevalent feature of the environment. Humans produce a lot of noise, from the rumble of traffic to the sound of musical instruments. From audible to inaudible, there are numerous distinct types of sound.

Whether a sound is pleasant or unpleasant depends on its source, type, volume, pitch, and intensity. Nevertheless, sound is a form of energy in motion. If the sonic properties are unpleasant, the resulting sounds may be regarded as pollutants.

Sound energy is a type of energy that is created when vibrations pass through a substance. These vibrations can travel through solids, liquids, and gases as waves, known as sound waves. Sound energy can be used in numerous ways, from communication to entertainment, even in medical applications.

One of the most common ways sound energy is used is by converting sound waves into electrical signals. Even though this science is constantly being developed, it is already widely implemented. This conversion allows for transmitting, storing, and manipulating sound information. Devices like microphones and speakers are common examples of this technology. Microphones convert sound waves into electrical signals, which can be stored and transmitted to other devices, while speakers convert electrical signals into sound waves, allowing us to audibly hear the information being communicated.

The conversion of sound energy into electrical signals is essential in many industries, from music and entertainment to medicine and telecommunications. For example, in the music industry, sound energy is used to create, record, and broadcast music. Similarly, in telecommunications, sound energy is used for voice communication over phone lines and internet connections.

In medicine, sound energy is used in diagnostic imaging technologies like ultrasound. Ultrasound employs high-frequency sound waves to create images of internal organs and structures, providing valuable information for medical diagnosis and treatment.

Potential Energy and Kinetic Energy

Although there are many different types of energy, there are two distinct states of energy in the universe: potential energy (energy existing in a reserved state) and kinetic energy (energy in motion).

Potential energy is that which has the capacity to work but isn't currently exerting force expressed as motion. In physics, the amount of energy transferred is used to calculate work. The technical definition of work is the act of moving something over a distance with the aid of an external force.

When placed at the top of a set of stairs, the Slinky's coiling spring illustrates potential energy. The spring isn't performing work until it is released. When the spring is activated, the slinky will climb down the stairs, transforming the energy expressed into kinetic energy. Kinetic energy is the force that propels motion. Sound energy is no exception and takes the form of kinetic or potential energy.

When applying these concepts to sound, playing a musical instrument actively creates sound waves. This is an expression of kinetic energy. However, when that same musical instrument is at rest, there is a complete transition to potential energy.

BRAIN WAVES

Each of us has felt the energizing sensation of being struck by a brain wave — that instance of fresh insight, a paradigm shift, or radical thought. And, usually, it seems to come from nowhere.

The exchange of signals between neurons in our brains is the basis for all our thoughts, feelings, and actions. There are billions of neurons in the brain, with each being connected to an average of thousands more. They communicate synaptically with one another via tiny electrical currents that travel along the neurons and across vast networks of brain circuitry. The simultaneous firing of these neurons is comparable to a wave rippling through the crowd at a sporting event. This coordinated electrical activity is what creates a brain wave event.

This simultaneous interaction between many neurons causes impulse energy that can be monitored and evaluated outside the brain. This cranial activity can be enhanced, investigated, and visualized by applying electrodes to the scalp linked to specialized medical equipment.

This process is known as electroencephalography, or EEG, essentially an electrical event brain graph.

The repetition rate of EEG brain waves is one means used to evaluate brain activity. When these impulse oscillations are measured, some have been found to occur at rates greater than 30 cycles per second and can reach up to 100 cycles per second. These cycles, also known as frequencies, are expressed in hertz in honor of the scientist, Heinrich Hertz, who first demonstrated the existence of electromagnetic waves.

Categorized in this way, there are five distinct types of brain waves, each represented by a different Greek letter. These various brain waves correspond to specific mental or emotional states. Although there are numerous other methods for studying brain waves, many experts in the discipline of neurofeedback rely on classifying brain oscillations into these five groups.

Gamma Waves

Gamma brain waves, which have a high frequency, comparable to a flute, are the fastest. Gamma waves fall between 32 and 100 Hz. They are linked to the simultaneous processing of information from different brain regions. Gamma brain waves transmit data quickly and quietly. Access to the gamma state requires a calm mind because it is the most subtle of the brain wave frequencies.

Gamma waves are found to be most active when experiencing universal love, altruism, and "higher virtues." Gamma waves are also produced at a frequency higher than neuronal firing, so their origin is unknown. Gamma rhythms are thought to affect perception and consciousness, and a higher concentration of gamma activity is associated with higher states of consciousness and spiritual awakening. Buddhist monks and other long-term meditators have been found to exhibit much more intense and consistent gamma brain wave activity.

Beta Waves

The highly engaged mind exhibits beta waves. Next to gamma waves, beta waves are the most rapid with a very small amplitude. Beta waves function in the frequency range above 12 Hz and typically fluctuate between 15 and 40 cycles per second.

Beta brain waves dominate during our normal waking state of consciousness when our attention is directed toward cognitive tasks and the outside world. The beta state is a fast mental activity that occurs when we are alert, focused, thinking critically, making decisions, or solving problems.

There are three levels of beta waves:

1. *Lo-Beta* (12–15 Hz): A fast idle or musing
2. *Beta* (15–22Hz): Active problem-solving or high engagement
3. *Hi-Beta* (22–38Hz): Very complex thought, assimilating new information, extreme anxiety or excitement

A person actively involved in conversation would be in a beta state; an individual engaged in a debate would be in high beta. While performing their duties, a public speaker, teacher, or talk show host would all be mentally functioning in the beta brain wave state.

Alpha Waves

In contrast to beta, which stands for arousal, alpha denotes the opposite. Alpha brain waves have a higher amplitude and are slower. The alpha band spans the frequency range of 8 to 12 Hz. These brain waves predominate during contemplative states and in some forms of meditation. They embody the capacity of being present – being "in the moment." Alpha is the state of rest for the brain. It supports the cognitive processes of learning, relaxation, and the fusion of the mind and body.

When someone takes some time to think or meditate, they are typically in an alpha state. A person who leaves a meeting to take a break or stroll through the garden would be in an alpha state.

Alpha is one of the most critical frequencies for the brain's ability to learn and apply knowledge, whether focusing in a classroom or concentrating at the workplace. When our alpha function operates within normal ranges, we experience positive moods, see the world plainly, and feel calm. Thinking or performing calculations will lower your alpha state; deep breathing and closing your eyes can raise it. Alpha-theta training has the effect of increasing sensation, abstract thought, and self-control.

Theta Brain Waves

Theta brain waves typically occur during sleep but can also be dominant during deep meditation. Theta activity is categorized as a slow state of being, with a frequency range of 3.5 to 7.5 Hz. It pertains to the subconscious mind and is a twilight state experienced between wakefulness and sleep. In theta, our senses become detached from the outside world and concentrate on sensory signals originating from within. Thus, it serves as an entryway to memory, intuition, and learning that is outside the scope of our ordinary conscious awareness. Theta waves are strong during inward focus, prayer, meditation, and spiritual awareness.

Theta brain wave states are frequently experienced by people who take breaks from tasks and start daydreaming; this is often brought on by the act of performing mundane or repetitive tasks. When someone is driving on a freeway and realizes they can't cognitively remember the last five miles, they've experienced the theta state.

Delta Brain Waves

Delta brain waves are the slowest brain waves recorded in humans. They are loud brain waves that deeply and quickly penetrate the skull like a drum beat. These brain waves operate on a frequency typically centered around 1.5 to 4 Hz. Deep, dreamless sleep conveys you to these slowest frequencies. Although delta brain waves lie in the lowest functional range, they never reach zero; if they did, you would literally be brain-dead.

Delta waves are attained during the most relaxed meditation and dreamless sleep states. Delta waves are the basis of empathy and suspend awareness of the outside world. The promotion of regeneration and healing in the delta state is evidence of the value of deep restorative sleep for maintaining the health of the body and mind.

THE INFLUENCE OF SOUND ON THE MIND AND BODY

The impact of sound on the human body has been recognized by scientists for hundreds of years. Studies have revealed that even inaudible high-frequency sounds can affect brain function. Similar to how shamanic chanting and drumming induce trance states, holistic healers also realize that different tonal frequencies can influence and even cause an altered state of human consciousness.

Healing and music have long been associated with both theology and medicine, dating back to ancient Greece. There are many ways to achieve sound frequency healing today, from participating in vibrational-acoustic therapies to listening to recordings of various binaural frequencies. Exposure to different frequencies can aid in treating mental health conditions like depression and anxiety, and genetic signaling can be used to encourage the body to combat physical illnesses.

Through music, sound frequencies can affect the body in ways that go beyond just healing. Music can evoke an emotional response in the body, resulting in everything from goosebumps or euphoria to a flood of therapeutic tears.

Hz Frequencies

Diverse frequencies and vibrations around us affect our bodies; some are beneficial, while others are particularly harmful. The human body operates between 62 and 72 Hz. With decreasing frequency, your body becomes weaker. If the frequency falls below 42 Hz, you have a significantly increased risk of developing cancer.

If you have been trying to eliminate negative energies, consider tuning into the frequency 528 Hz. Tuning into this frequency, your body is doing more than just letting you unwind. The balance and recovery of your body's cells are encouraged by the

528 Hz frequency. It is also maintained that subjecting yourself to this specific frequency facilitates your endocrine system to lower cortisol levels, resulting in a stress-free body and mind. Reducing stress can be as simple as listening to music or other sounds whose core frequency focuses at 528 Hz. Below are additional healing frequencies you may benefit from:

- *40 Hz:* This frequency stimulates memory by interacting with gamma brain waves.
- *174 Hz:* This is a solfeggio frequency, which is regarded as sacred music that encourages meditation.
- *285 Hz:* This frequency is useful for the healing of bodily wounds such as cuts and burns.
- *396 Hz:* This frequency is used to get rid of anxiety and other unpleasant emotions.
- *417 Hz:* This frequency is used to cleanse the body and mind of old trauma.

Binaural Beats

The science behind binaural beats follows these premises. When a sound frequency is played in the right ear, a single tone can be heard. When a similar but slightly different sound frequency is played in the left ear, a single tone will also be heard there. However, when these two tones are played simultaneously, your brain "hears" the vibrato between them as a distinct beat. It is this interaction and how our brain interprets what it is experiencing that is known as a binaural beat.

For instance, you might introduce a sound in your left ear that is 200 Hz in pitch while presenting a sound in your right ear at

210 Hz. Your brain, however, gradually synchronizes with the difference (10 Hz). Instead of hearing two distinct tones, you hear a tone at a frequency of 10 Hz in addition to the two varying tones delivered to each ear respectively.

Harmonically incorporating the concept of binaural beats into music allows you to subtly direct your brain wave activity to a desired state. The binaural beat is still present and functioning whether or not your ears can hear it. Suppose you regularly listen to binaural beats that promote deep meditation (theta and delta brain waves). In this case, your brain's two hemispheres will function in balance and harmony.

Binaural beats have been demonstrated to aid in promoting the meditative state, lower anxiety, improve moods, stimulate creativity, strengthen cognitive function, and increase focus and memory retention. With listening to binaural beats, your brain activity synchronizes with the frequency established by the beat. This is referred to as the frequency-following effect. This means that you can train your brain to achieve a particular state of consciousness using binaural beats.

Solfeggio Frequencies

The solfeggio frequencies are a part of the ancient six-tone scale, which is believed to include sacred music like the well-known and stunning Gregorian chants. These distinctive tones and chants are intended to bestow spiritual blessings when played harmoniously. Every solfeggio tone contains the frequencies required for energy balancing and maintaining the ideal state of harmony between the spirit, mind, and body.

Solfeggio includes the technique of solmization, which is the use of sol-fa syllables to note scale tones. Another well-known application of solfeggio is as a singing exercise in which syllables are used rather than words. Solfeggio comes in two varieties:

1. Fixed Do

These pitches are predetermined and never change. Do is always C natural, and it then moves up from there. Simply put, Do, Re, Mi, Fa, Sol, La, Si, Do are always C, D, E, F, G, A, B, and C.

2. Movable Do

In this application, the movement changes depending on the key signature of the musical piece. Despite using the same Do, Re, Mi, Fa, Sol, La, Si, and Do syllables, their designated pitches vary to match the root pitch. Consequently, Do is C if you are in the key of C, while Do is D if you are in the key of D. In essence, it is a note naming convention referencing each element according to its relative pitch, with Do serving as the major tonic.

Below are the fundamental frequencies used in solfeggio.

- 174 Hz for reducing pain and anxiety
- 285 Hz for healing tissues and organs
- 396 Hz for releasing oneself from guilt and fear
- 417 Hz for promoting change and fixing adverse circumstances

- 528 Hz for wonders and transformations, including DNA repair
- 639 Hz for reconnection and relationships
- 741 Hz for finding answers and self-expression
- 852 Hz for rejoining a spiritual hierarchy
- 963 Hz for creating space for interconnectedness, harmony, and unity.

While solfeggio frequencies are rarely heard in popular music, they are frequently employed in sound healing techniques and new-age music to encourage spiritual growth and self-healing.

Sine Wave Voice Harmonics

Relationship and proportion are the two key components of harmonies. These harmonies are produced using straightforward mathematical ratios to establish pleasant interactions between sounds. As a result, we have discovered that numerous harmonies can be used for healing because of their clear mathematical relationship and because they promote a positive state of being. Such harmonics produce an ethereal sense of health, balance, tranquility, and beauty.

The passage of sound through space can be understood geometrically in a variety of ways. For example, we can think of sound as a sine wave with peaks and valleys. One complete cycle of a periodic sine wave consists of one full peak and valley of the corresponding waveform. The number of cycles a sound wave completes each second is expressed as its hertz value.

When two sound waves with different frequencies repeatedly intersect respective to time, they are both geometrically and audibly harmonic. The simpler the mathematical ratio, or in other words, the more frequently musical tones complete their cycle at the same point, the more harmonically pleasing the sound when played simultaneously.

Interestingly, as the proportions become more complex, our ears also discern the decline in harmony. This suggests that as sound enters our ears and is converted into an electrical signal in the brain, we perceive elevated beauty in the simple proportion and relationship of the two sounds. This actually nourishes us neurologically.

When the sounds interplay with each other less frequently, they grow ominous and more discordant. These dissonant waveforms, which invoke a different neurological response, can also be used therapeutically to clear, dismiss, or resolve sensory states.

SOUND AND HEALING

Sonic vibrational stimuli influencing the body is a lengthy operational process. It enters through the ear's nerves, moves to the brain, and then spreads throughout the body. The body reacts in response to the vibrations it experiences. Using sound for wellness is a great way to connect the mind and body and encourage healing. Sound healing operates in levels. It starts with emotional healing, moves on to mental healing, and finally progresses to physical healing.

Sound Baths

In a sound bath, participants are bathed in sound waves during a meditative session. Several instruments, including gongs, singing bowls, various percussive instruments, chimes, rattles, tuning forks, and even human voices, can be implemented to produce these waves. Instead of having a memorable melody or rhythm like you would hear at a symphony or rock concert, the music is a carefully chosen wash of instruments and voices with pronounced resonance and overtones.

The intent is that the participant's energy be altered and balanced. It necessitates that they do not get hooked on a tune or beat during the sound bath. You want to avoid making the rhythm or melody repetitive or predictable because you don't wish the participant's brain to recognize a repeated beat. Instead, the goal is for the individual to be released internally and for the brain to let go of traditional stimuli.

Sound Meditation

Sound has long been associated with healing and meditation. Sound meditation incorporates the use of sound and music to concentrate and encourage more profound contemplations. Many different cultures, religions, and mystic traditions still use this age-old custom. Music has multiple dimensions, connecting various brain regions and enabling reflection independent of thought.

Although it can be used with any genre of sound, the most effective sound sources include singing bowls, gongs, and chanting. The purpose of the sound is to help you focus on the here and now and let go of distractions.

A powerful technique for promoting relaxation and stress relief is sound meditation. It can also improve sleep quality and raise feelings of well-being. Additionally, using sound during introspection can help you focus and better understand and appreciate reality.

Sonopuncture/Osteophony/Diaphony

It has been observed that applying an ultrasound stimulus to the acupuncture meridian system is safe and effective for many typical clinical conditions for which there are limited treatments. The use of tuning forks is an excellent and efficient way to apply sound to the body, including the acupoints, trigger and reflex points, bone, muscle, and tendons, to help tonify or disperse Qi (life energy). This is implemented to help relieve pain and harmonize the body at the cellular level.

Tuning forks produce pure sounds. Their designs are explicitly modeled to generate pure sine waves devoid of harmonics (overtones). After striking the fork, any overtones quickly dissipate, leaving only the fundamental pitch to transmit the vibrational energy. Each fork's specific frequency is clearly stamped into the body and can be used in numerous ways.

Maintaining homeostasis is essential for physical, mental, and spiritual healing. The use of various forks affects our biological clocks and circadian rhythms. This enables us to align with nature's cycles, achieving and sustaining the desirable balance of life.

Tuning forks with high vibration and resonance are linked to the body's natural frequencies and support them. The fork's vibrational sonic waves penetrate the body deeply along energy pathways, affecting human physiology and permitting access to our sense of equilibrium, space, memory, and healing. This mechanism energizes and harmonizes the physical energy field of the body to support recovery and inner harmony, thus integrating body, mind, and spirit, enhancing remembrance and regeneration.

1. Sonopuncture

This new age healing process involves applying tuning forks to the body's reflex points, including acupuncture points, meridian points, hand and foot reflexology points, spinal reflex points, Shiatsu points, and all other noted therapeutic foci.

2. Osteophony

Osteophony is a medical term used to describe the abnormal sounds or noises heard during the physical examination of bones. These sounds are produced due to changes in the density or structure of the bone and can be indicative of underlying pathologies such as fractures, tumors, or osteoporosis. Osteophony can be detected through various means such as percussion, auscultation, and palpation, and can aid in the diagnosis and management of bone-related disorders. Applying tuning forks to the articulations and other skeletal components are one of the more typical techniques. Bones are the most efficient vibration transmitters of any human anatomy.

3. Diaphony

Whereas osteophony pertains to the bones, diaphony is a medical term referring to the perception of sound transmission through tissues, such as the lungs or the abdomen. It is commonly used to assess the quality and intensity of respiratory or bowel sounds during a physical examination. Diaphony can be detected through various techniques, such as auscultation and percussion. It can help diagnose underlying pathologies such as lung consolidation or bowel obstruction. Diaphony is a valuable tool for clinicians in identifying and managing respiratory and gastrointestinal disorders. Furthermore, holistically, this methodology refers to tuning forks providing evaluation and support for the aura, chakras (the body's electromagnetic energy centers and fields), and subtle bodies' energy fields and energy centers.

HEALING SOUND INSTRUMENTS

Using sound as a healing medium has been practiced for thousands of years in nearly every culture and tradition, from the Aboriginal use of the yidaki (or didgeridoo) to treat physical ailments to the ancient oriental gong used for spiritual attunement.

The vibrations transmitted can impact us at the cellular level, depending on the instrument. Some instruments significantly assist us in transitioning from beta brain wave patterns, which are linked to focus, anxiety, and the fight-or-flight response, to calmer frequencies such as alpha, theta, and even delta brain waves. These brain waves are associated with the trance (delta), the meditative (theta), and the relaxation (alpha) states of consciousness.

1. Hammered Dulcimer

The hammered dulcimer has a breathtaking sound. Except for being played like a drum, making this a percussive instrument, the hammered dulcimer is similar to an open piano or a harp. It is also one of the most widely used sound therapy tools for unwinding and easing the symptoms of stress and anxiety.

2. Gong

Meditation gongs, one of the earliest instruments for sound healing, are reputed to have the power to rebalance the body, mind, and spirit. The gong has been used since 4000 BC for practices like chakra balancing, yoga, and meditation. They are frequently employed in Buddhist sound meditations as well. They produce a full, resonant sound that we can use to maintain focus during meditation.

3. Wind Chimes/Koshi

Wind chimes can be traced back to ancient Rome, India, and China. Wind chimes are frequently used in feng shui to maximize the flow of Qi because they effectively transmit gorgeous celestial sounds and timbres. Due to their relaxing, characteristic sound, millions of people hang wind chimes outside their homes. A Koshi is a name for the conventional variety of wind chimes used in sound healing. These instruments are tuned specifically for use in sound therapy.

4. Pan Flute

Pan flutes date back more than 6,000 years. They are typically made of wood, ivory, and bamboo, and their use is widespread in South American nations like Bolivia, Peru, and Ecuador. Folk music frequently incorporates the pan flute's sweet, mellow, and calming melodies.

5. Singing Bowl

Since the 12th century, singing bowls have been used for meditation techniques throughout Asia. They are also traditionally found in Tibetan temples and monasteries. In addition to being used for sound healing therapy, singing bowls are now frequently used in spiritual ceremonies, yoga, and traditional and modern meditation practices.

With respect for all sound healing devices, singing bowls are arguably the most effective. They produce sound frequencies that open and balance the seven chakras, promoting overall well-being. These characteristics make singing bowls largely the most suitable sound healing instruments.

6. Handpan

The handpan is a harmonic, spherical-shaped instrument typically with eight different playing surfaces. Each handpan can be manufactured to a customized harmonic tuning. This instrument was created by two Swiss inventors, Felix Rohner and Sabina Schärer, in 2000. Depending on how it is played, the handpan can produce sounds similar to those of a steelpan or a singing bowl. It can be used to support meditation or simply to calm and center the mind.

7. Tuning Fork

Tuning forks are both an instrument and tool used in sound healing therapy to assist the body in regaining its natural tuning by employing extremely precise frequencies. The forks are applied by experts in a manner resembling acupuncture to specific body regions. Having the tools to apply such precise frequencies to very specific body structures afford the practitioner tremendous latitude for releasing somatic energy blockages.

8. Didgeridoo

The didgeridoo is an Australian instrument that has been around for approximately 1,500 years and was traditionally used in Aboriginal ceremonies. It is constructed from wood and painted with traditional designs. The didgeridoo is played by blowing through one end to produce its deep, characteristic resonance. Its application for music therapy is to clear emotional and energetic stagnation along with support for meditation and mind-body healing.

9. Kalimba

Kalimbas, also referred to as Mbiras or thumb pianos, have their roots in Africa and have existed for a very long time. The Kalimba, often made of wood with metal keys, sounds similar to that of a harp or a Hang and is easily played. In Zimbabwe, the Kalimba has been used to treat both physical and mental illnesses.

10. Djembe

The djembe is a drum that is native to West Africa and is constructed out of wood, rope, and goat skin. It is frequently employed to create trance-like states of altered consciousness as well as to relieve stress and anxiety.

11. Rainstick

Rainsticks, thought to have been created by the Aztecs, are usually made from dried cacti bodies with items like small pebbles inserted inside. As the name suggests, rainsticks are used to promote calm and peace by producing a sound resembling that of rain.

12. Native American Flute

The Native American flute is a magnificent instrument with a riveting sound that transports us to a more archaic state of being. Its incredibly calming and relaxing sound has been demonstrated to lower stress, slow the heartbeat, stabilize blood pressure, and lessen symptoms of depression and anxiety. Sound healing therapy employs the flute's sonic character to create inner balance by returning the body and mind to their harmonious states.

THE HEALING GUITAR

Undoubtedly there are innumerable accounts that attest to the benefits of using sound and music in a manner that promotes wellness and improves the quality of daily life.

In my own experience, I often had the opportunity to observe the life of a young woman, presently in her teens, who was diagnosed with Rett Syndrome. This disease severely restricts an individual's capacity to express their thoughts, feelings, and emotions. Although I am fully aware of the physical constraints that prevent my young friend from expressing her inner life as freely as the rest of us, I do not doubt that she possesses any less of these humanities. Her parents' excellent care of their daughter has granted her more opportunity than most with her condition. As a result of their devotion to her and their tenacious efforts to help her, she had the privilege to walk for a short while despite the doctors' predictions that she would never be able to do so.

Regardless of the circumstances, little is as heartwarming as witnessing her blossom with life when her parents take out a guitar and sing to her. Even though she cannot sing herself and will never be expected to learn to play the guitar, her parents' willingness and enthusiasm to share their own songs allow her to express that she is very much alive and a part of that music.

The powerful and inspiring possibilities of sound and music are limitless. At this time, I admonish you to reflect on your own experiences when you have witnessed the simple virtues of a song wonderfully transforming you or a loved one; remember, savor, relive those moments. Consider that you have the opportunity to consistently enrich your ordinary days with the influence of sound and music.

4

SOUND AS THERAPY

A person does not hear sound only through the ears; he hears sound through every pore of the body. It permeates the entire being, and according to its particular influence, either slows or quickens the rhythm of the blood circulation; it either awakens or soothes the nervous system.

— HAZRAT INAYAT KHAN

MUSIC THERAPY

The powerful therapeutic qualities of music afford music therapy to effectively improve a person's well-being. It is a technique of expressive arts therapy that incorporates music to enhance and preserve a person's physical, psychological, and social well-being; it encompasses various activities, including but not limited to singing, playing an instrument, and listening to music.

A qualified therapist facilitates this professional therapy, which is becoming more frequently used in hospitals, rehab facilities, schools, prisons, nursing homes, and hospices.

Music has the power to evoke positive emotions and activate the reward centers of the brain. The diverse nature of music makes it possible to treat both physical and psychological needs. In some cases, the therapeutic use of music has aided patients in ways that other types of therapy have been notably limited, eliciting reactions and stimulating responses less readily seen through more conventional types of treatment. When people have trouble expressing themselves verbally, music therapy has been demonstrated to pique a patient's interest and engagement more than other long-standing traditional treatment methods. It has further been established that prior musical training and experience aren't required for a patient to enjoy its benefits.

Through the use of music therapy interventions, a wide range of healthcare and educational goals can be met, including fostering wellness, managing stress, relieving pain, expressing feelings, improving memory and concentration, facilitating communication, and assisting with physical rehabilitation.

Mental Health

Structured use of binaural beats is an emerging therapy technique for treating a wide range of mental health-related problems. The effectiveness of binaural beats is conditional with respect to the duration, frequency, and timing of aural exposure to them.

Because binaural beats adhere to a specific sound pattern that evolves over time, binaural beats must be listened to from the beginning linearly without skipping segments to achieve the greatest cognitive benefits.

1. Anxiety and stress

Recognizing anxiety for what it is and determining what most effectively helps manage it are two of the main objectives of regulating anxiety. Binaural beats are sometimes used by therapists as a mindfulness training tool, along with other practices in the form of breathing exercises and guided imagery, which have proven successful in reducing stress in patients. Due to how our brains are wired to respond to sound, receptive music therapies can serve as a cue for pausing and reflecting on our feelings.

Study resources indicate that following 40 minutes of exposure to delta frequency (2.5 Hz) binaural beats, healthy participants' anxiety lessens. When implementing these measures for one's own benefit, it is best to experiment with a few different frequencies in the delta range to determine which is most helpful for the individual. By doing this, it is possible to identify the ideal frequency that best reduces anxiety for a specific person.

2. Sleep

Up to one-third of adults experience insomnia, making sleep issues disturbingly prevalent and concerning. There are numerous potential causes for sleep disorders, including stress, mental health issues, sleep and lifestyle habits, and specific medications. Furthermore, the compounded sleep crisis of a combination of any of the conditions listed above is additionally disconcerting.

As with anxiety, new research shows that binaural beats also may aid in treating insomnia and speeding the process of falling asleep for people with healthy sleep patterns.

Typically, frequencies between 4 and 8 Hz are effective because they represent the change from theta to delta or awake to asleep states. Applying this aural input similar to sleep-related brain activity promoting sleep suggests that brain functionality can actively be regulated with acoustic signals. Binaural beats additionally can be implemented to lengthen stage three sleep, the state of deep sleep most attributed to waking up feeling rested.

3. Memory and Attention

According to mental-audio correlation studies, binaural beats improve reasoning, comprehension, and goal-oriented behavior by assisting the brain in organizing and retaining information that has been gathered and stored throughout the day.

Cranial neurons can be stimulated by binaural beats, resulting in a broad array of feelings and behaviors. One beneficial application for this knowledge is that a person's brain in the alpha state will function at its peak, allowing them to focus on and solidify demanding memory and learning tasks.

To use binaural beats for concentration, audio signals must be listened to at low volume. The brain can more easily enter the focus-oriented alpha state when exposed to a frequency differential between 8 and 12 Hz. Doing this allows an individual to maintain expanded levels of focus, even training oneself to enter and take advantage of the super alpha learning state. However, one should note that it is best to use these heightened focus methods only for a short time per each session.

Physical Health

Sound healing uses frequency to balance and harmonize the body's vibrations during treatment. The sound properties selected incorporate frequencies that slow brain waves to a healing stage. The patient usually lies down on the floor and relaxes while the therapist plays various musical instruments. The sound produced by these instruments gives the impression that the listener is bathed in vibrations from many sound sources. Sound therapy takes advantage of various tools, including but not limited to Tibetan singing bowls, tuning forks, and a myriad of traditional instruments.

Sound therapy has been used successfully to treat numerous conditions, including hypertension, depression, sleep disorders, and autism. According to music therapy studies, listening to music can lower stress levels, strengthen the immune system, and have anti-inflammatory effects. Less stress and anxiety allow the body to maintain healthy cellular activity and defend against disease, key elements to promoting and sustaining homeostasis - the balance of life.

In addition to helping people relax, sound therapy helps people break through other physical health barriers. It regulates hormones and stimulates endocrine gland activity. It additionally lowers blood pressure and assists in clearing out toxins from the body. Still, most importantly, it aligns the chakras, which regulate the energy systems supporting these physical entities.

1. Yogic chanting and "Om"-ing

Chanting can be used as a meditation tool and a way to keep one's health and well-being in check. Chanting helps with heart rate regulation, blood pressure reduction, circulation enhancement, endorphin production, and metabolism support.

Chanting reduces stress because it sharpens the mind. For instance, the mantra "om" is frequently regarded as paramount in yoga because it fosters profound mental clarity and makes one feel more connected to a higher power.

2. Classical music

Classical music has been attributed the ability to expedite the rate of synaptic connections being formed in the brain. Along with fostering creativity and enhancing learning, this music genre moderates physical conditions like high blood pressure, anxiety, and muscle tension.

3. Humming

Humming is a simple and enjoyable activity that can offer a variety of benefits for your mental and physical health. When you hum, you create a vibration in your throat that can produce a calming effect on your body and mind. This supports relieving stress, anxiety, even reducing blood pressure. Humming also increases the body's natural production of nitric oxide which is known to have many additional positive effects on your cardiovascular health. Furthermore, humming can improve your breathing and vocal control along with boosting your mood and energy levels. Possibly one of the most surprising benefits is that it aids in maintaining a healthy and clear sinus system.

4. Tuning forks

Tuning forks were initially employed to adjust musical instruments to the right pitch. Orthopedists have since started using tuning forks to locate stress fractures in large bones. Tuning fork vibrations are used by sound therapists to direct more energy toward various internal organs they are endeavoring to heal. Positive vibes help with relaxation, nervous system balance, and an increase in stamina.

5. Singing bowls

Singing bowls can be made of metal or quartz crystal. The functional tones are created by striking the edge of the bowl with a wooden striker or felt-padded mallet. A wooden striker will produce a metallic, high-pitched sound. A felt-padded mallet, on the other hand, will create a richer, kinder, warmer tone. The ensuing vibrations and tones cause the heart rate, brain waves, and breathing to slow down, inducing a profound sense of calm and general well-being.

Achieving Brain Wave States

Neurological studies suggest that regulated sound waves can positively impact our brain waves and assist us in managing a variety of health problems. This is significant because occasionally less desirable brain states are induced by sound waves from our environment, and binaural beats can be used to offset the influence of those unwanted stimuli. Science offers an effortless way to facilitate changes in brain wave activity through audio stimulation (specific tones and rhythms used with a headset) that takes advantage of binaural beats. This method, known as brain wave entrainment, is one approach people incorporate to manipulate their brain activity to achieve a desired mental state.

As alpha waves are associated with feelings of relaxation, achieving them is the most common goal of brain entrainment. Most people can produce these mental frequencies simply by closing their eyes while taking slow deep breaths. Still, certain individuals are not able to naturally generate them at all.

The entrainment process coaxes brain waves to match the frequency of an external stimulus, such as a binaural beat. It regulates brain regions that would otherwise fire at discordant rates. The idea is that once your brain starts to synchronize at the targeted rate, you'll begin to exhibit the associated mental state.

Inducing gamma or beta waves in your brain, can help you pay attention when you need to study for a test or concentrate at work. On the opposite end of the spectrum, those who struggle with insomnia may attempt to impose a theta or delta wave to regulate their mental state to aid with sleeping. One can look up "delta binaural beats" or "alpha binaural beats" on YouTube or many other music services to readily find specific binaural beats tracks to instill the desired frame of mind. If you find binaural beats too repetitious or dull, other music sources are available which are also designed to achieve particular mental states.

Brain entrainment can be a quick and efficient treatment for people struggling with anxiety, pain, discomfort, sleep disorders, or focus issues. This resource might also be worth noting as a helpful tool for stress management or meditation exercise enhancement for anyone needing a little additional help relaxing or clearing the mind.

At-Home Sound Bath

Taking a sound bath can help you relax completely. The object here is to achieve the alpha brain state, better known as relaxed consciousness, by immersing oneself in a sonic environment. These corresponding brain wave frequencies are linked to a calm, clear, meditative state of mind. The same frequency range also assists with lowering stress, anxiety, and insomnia. This state of being can furthermore benefit those in pain or experiencing trauma.

To create your own personal sound bath, use a Tibetan singing bowl. Suppose you don't have access to a singing bowl; in that case, you can listen to online sources, preferably wearing headphones, but standard speakers are acceptable. Give yourself plenty of room and time.

When you are ready to start, lie down in a comfortable position. Before making any sounds, hold the singing bowl while settling on an intended focus for your experience. Start inhaling deeply and slowly into your abdomen. After that, use a mallet to gently tap the bowl's edge. As the note slowly fades, let your attention be drawn to the sound and to the focus you have set — inhaling what you wish for and exhaling to let go.

Feel the ground beneath you supporting you. Keep striking the bowl throughout your meditation; a slow rhythm is encouraged to help maintain a relaxed body and mind. As you progress, trusting that you are in a safe environment, let go and relax completely, close your eyes, and drift away.

The singing bowl's tone induces complete silence from all other sounds and voices within you, filling your body with unified sound to help you regain your equilibrium. Take additional deep breaths allowing yourself to be guided by the instrument's high-frequency healing as you transition from the initial alpha state to a deep theta-meditative journey — the ideal way to unwind, relax and rejuvenate.

You'll experience a journey through the sound. Everybody has different experiences, so if you discover yourself getting sidetracked by a thought, try acknowledging it and letting it go rather than getting hung up on it. Allow yourself to savor whatever is beckoning to you, sit with that emotion, and then let it go.

SOUND AND MUSIC THERAPY IN EVERYDAY LIFE

How often have you walked around wearing your headphones or having your Bluetooth speaker connected, contemplating what music would best suit your mood at that particular time? Does this cause you to perceive your surroundings differently? How does this influence your experience?

Early man first used music as a form of communication, stemming from the need to communicate vocally. Since then, people have progressively learned to use music for socializing, creativity, and healing.

Born in 570 BC, over 2500 years ago, Greek philosopher Pythagoras recommended musical scales in various modes to treat a variety of illnesses. According to a notable biblical account, the young Israelite David soothed King Saul with the lyre nearly 500 years prior to this because it relieved the monarch from being taunted by an evil spirit. Some have hypothesized that this evil spirit may be equated to depression or anxiety in the modern world.

Sea shanties or musical chants like the traditional "Drunken Sailor," which provided rhythmic support for organizing, motivating, and sustaining effort, were once the embodiment of sailors making their way around the globe. This allowed them to synergistically lift heavy anchor lines, raise enormous sails, load and unload cargo, and row in a synchronized manner. This coordinated effort was made possible by music. If they hadn't been able to work together to complete this task using the power of rhythmic music, chaos would have ensued. Their efforts would have become cumbersome.

These ancient musical applications paved the way for how we use music to regulate our bodies and minds today. We react to music in one way or another from the moment of our conception until the moment we take our final breath. This might be because we are born with an innate rhythm already inside us: our heartbeat. Or perhaps there is a deeper source.

In the most trying times of our lives, the concepts of music therapy aid in our healing and success. We listen to music to get pumped up, we find inner peace, empathize with others, and give our emotions validation and release. We are inextricably linked to music; it can be heard in our breathing, speech, movement, and heartbeat. Even in our speaking voices, there is tone and melody.

We are all born with the ability to react to music. Despite illness or impairment, this response prevails. Music therapists are firm believers in music's capacity to bridge racial, cultural, and linguistic divides without using words. When it comes to improving our mental health, music therapy can act as the link between illness and health, discomfort and comfort, misperception and understanding, and resistance and acceptance.

Sound has a remarkable ability to affect the brain. The brain is stimulated and calmed by music, and it aids in detecting patterns and organizing brain states. Numerous cognitive and physical conditions can be treated with music therapy using the principles of sound, knowledge of how different types of sound interact with the brain and body, and solid scientific research in this field of study.

We can observe from MRI scans that it directly affects the regions of the brain responsible for attention, memory, coordination, and emotional processing. Life skills like communication, interaction, spontaneity, flexibility, self-expression, and self-confidence are all enhanced by music therapy.

We all listen to music virtually every day in an effort to comfort ourselves, relax, and find inspiration. As a healing aid, music is enticing, enjoyable, nonintrusive, and is deeply meaningful. We all find warmth from this familiar and invaluable resource.

Self-Healing

Music unquestionably affects our mood; innately possessing the power to dramatically alter our dispositions. Slow, minor-chord music can make us feel melancholy and nostalgic while conjuring up possibly lamentable memories. We only have to listen to one sad song to succumb to being miserable. Major chords, a more rapid tempo, and upbeat tones have the opposite effect; they uplift, energize, and encourage us to move forward - to take action. The truth is that music speaks to our feelings instantaneously and is genuinely the language of emotion.

The sounds we are surrounded by can quickly become a constant noise that impairs our ability to listen and maintain concentration. Noise all too often wears us out... exhausts us... stresses us out. Some examples of external sources of noise pollution are busy roads and highways, aircraft, motorcycles, railroads, factories, industrial settings, construction sites, and loud concerts, as well as internal sources like TVs, loudspeakers, stereo systems, mixers, air conditioners, and many other items we use on a daily basis. As soon as we become aware of the noise, we have the option to choose how to shield ourselves from its damaging influence. We can retain our equilibrium and lower our stress levels by minimizing their effects as much as possible.

Nature

One of the great opportunities we have at our disposal is that we can choose to listen to sounds that are healing. Instead of constantly feeding our minds on the negativity of current events via every news channel, etc., nature is a great place to find sounds that are calming and restoring. It dramatically increases our vitality and benefits both our physical and mental well-being. Nature-based activities lower blood pressure, ease stress and anxiety, calm the mind, and foster a positive, vibrant outlook on life. Accessing nature and hearing its sounds may not always be available depending on our living circumstances. However, in today's technologically advanced world, you can access a wide range of high-quality nature sounds from countless online sources and enter an alternative world as easily as closing your eyes.

• Forest wind

The wind's sound is calming and unwinding; it lacks any obtrusive or antagonistic tones that might annoy or ruin the experience. Taking pleasure in the sound of the wind can calm and lessen stress and anxiety. Additionally, it imparts fresh vitality and a cheerful disposition.

Imagine being surrounded by tall, silent pine trees in a forest. Take a moment to pause and remain still. Respond to the sounds, allowing their rhythm and vibration to reverberate in your soul. Observe and listen to the wind as it whispers in the branches of the trees and blows through the tree crowns, creating the most remarkable, calming sound that one can hope to experience. It seems the trees are speaking, imparting ancient knowledge with magical healing properties that they have preserved for centuries yet share with any that seek for it.

• Rain

Raindrop sounds and rhythm have a calming and soothing effect. It is a great way to ground yourself and feel comforted.

Take a moment to picture yourself strolling through a lovely, well-groomed park. You feel a single water drop land on your arm. Another follows on your cheek. You quickly look around for cover before taking shelter beneath a large willow tree. You close your eyes and quietly sit there as you listen to the surreal sound of rain. Every raindrop makes a distinct splattering sound as it hits the leaves at first, followed by a light, jovial pitter-patter. After some time, the rain becomes more intense and comes down in sheets, dousing the ground around you as well as the nearby leaves with water. But it doesn't intrude on you. It's one of those harmless showers that doesn't interfere with anything but brings a renewed freshness to all the life surrounding you. You feel at ease and drowsy listening to the raindrops' constant rustling. It seems to have the cadence of a comforting lullaby.

• Birdsong

Early in the morning, listening to birdsong can bring joy and set the mood for a good day. Simply take it in while sitting still and listening with a light, open heart. Solo performers might enter the stage and deliver beautiful arias before moving on to allow the next feathered performer to take the stage. Every performer gets to shine at some point. Yet the blending of their song is just as wonderfully harmonious. The result is an incredible sound and a beautiful spring dawn melody that will uplift your spirits as the birds combine styles, tones, and rhythm.

• Sea waves

There is something marvelously calming about the sound of the ocean, the salty air, and the warmth of the sand between your toes. The sound of waves crashing instills powerful inspiration, creativity, and insight while concurrently reducing any sense of stress and healing brokenness.

Visualize a sea with dynamic waves that crash against the shore. At first, nothing else can be heard over the thunderous sound of the waves. It may ostensibly sound irate, crashing hard against the coast. Initially, you might feel intimidated, but as its call holds you longer, you are immersed in the environment, beginning to enjoy the intense sound of the breakers, and discover a melody and rhythm in that sound — partly monotonous, but seemingly alive with its continuous flow that leaves you feeling content, at ease, and inspired.

Voice

People frequently underestimate the healing potential of the human voice as a sound healing tool. Even though it is the most versatile tool we have at our disposal, our voice could be far more abundantly utilized as an instrument, so it is critical to bear in mind its full potential. Vocal toning and chanting are two basic ways to begin using your voice to support healing and general welfare.

• Vocal toning

This technique can lull a person into a state of deep relaxation.

Take a moment to center yourself, take a few deep breaths, and increase awareness of your surroundings as well as yourself within them. Focus on your breathing. Close your eyes and your mouth. Start humming a low pitch. Allow the resonance of the sound to be felt throughout your body. After humming for a few minutes (ideally five), notice how you feel.

Due to the way we cognitively process sound in the brain, low pitches tend to relax the nervous system. You receive an internal massage from keeping the sound inside your body, which aids in maintaining your focus and may also relieve upper-back, neck, and shoulder tension. Being present in the moment through awareness helps reduce stress and anxiety.

Studies have shown that a brief singing session significantly increases immunoglobulin A (an antibody). Again, as always, it is inspiring to know that something as simple as singing is not only pleasantly enjoyable but has added benefits for your health.

• **Chanting**

Essentially all cultures have used chanting for thousands of years to elevate the spirit and awaken specific archetypal energies within oneself. Select a concise, repetitive chant that is simple to learn so that you do not have to expend effort trying to remember it. It can come from any tradition, but it should be one you are comfortable with, which leaves you feeling at ease.

Chanting raises the physiology's overall vibration. Lose yourself in the chant by opening your heart and throat and chanting with your entire body. You are ultimately chanting for the essence of life within.

The chant "Om" is well-liked and powerful. Breathe in deeply. When you exhale, chant the mantra "Om." When you run out of breath, take an additional deep breath and continue the chant. Continue for another two to three minutes at your own pace.

MHz

As already discussed in some detail in this book, MHz healing is one of the simplest ways to access the brain through the body, avoiding our conscious inner critic and focusing solely on the specific regions of concern that require attention. Numerous tracks on YouTube and other pertinent websites exist for exercising these practices.

Using MHz frequencies before or after social interactions can help with social anxiety. They can also aid in recovery following daily activities, physical workouts, and housework. An additional application is selecting an appropriate MHz sound file attuned for night use. Use a timer on the player device set to end after a reasonable period of time before turning in for the night. The optimal time chosen may require some experimentation, but the timer prevents sleep from being interrupted. This procedure can help you experience a restful night's sleep and feel much better when you wake the next day.

EXERCISE

Experience sound healing for yourself at the conclusion of this chapter: Select a soothing sound source from nearly any music website or YouTube, such as an MHz tone, binaural beat, solfeggio, or another similar sound source, and play it before bed. For the best results, use headphones, but again speakers are acceptable. Experiment. Try listening for 30 minutes before going to bed; 20 minutes, an hour. Then compare the results using the timer method described in the previous section (MHz).

Note your findings; what methods work best, which don't, and which sound files are most effective. Record as much detail as possible so that you can recreate the most effective sources and methods. Create playlists to avoid getting tired of repetition to continue cultivating the benefits.

Then expand on these concepts. Explore and discover what sounds and music put you in a good mood for the day to face work or school. You likely already have your favorite playlists for your workouts; expand on them to include your post-workout cool-down.

How do you react to social events, visits from relatives and friends? Can you incorporate music into the routine to improve the outcome during and after these events? This list goes on. You get the idea, so let's stop here. You can take as much advantage and benefit from this nearly inexhaustible resource as you choose. Most of all, enjoy the journey; sound encompasses entire worlds.

5

SOUND HEALING FOR THE BODY

Sound is medicine. Use it wisely.

— MICHAEL BETTINE

SOUND HEALING FOR PHYSICAL WELL-BEING

Regarding your physical well-being, checking your overall health status before pursuing more complex therapies is crucial. Always examine the fundamentals: your diet, hydration, gut health, exercise, sleep, inflammation, and infection. Address any concerns that may be out of balance or harmony. However, if you are uncertain of any of your symptoms, always seek the advice and guidance of a licensed medical professional.

Sound therapy will not conflict with any other medications or treatments; on the contrary, it most often will synergistically strengthen them. The sound of instruments and voices helps to release energy tangles and harmonize the body as a whole. The vibrations move throughout the body and widen energy channels, enhancing circulation and releasing feel-good endorphins. These sound vibrations help regulate brain wave signaling to elevate mood, which promotes healing throughout your body.

Aches and Pains

Brain function can directly and easily be stimulated through sound. One method to activate the entire brain using sound therapy implements enhanced high frequencies and heavily filtered classical music. Regular Sonic exposure of this nature, which reconnects pertinent brain regions, delivers the signal mechanism that the brain requires to stop sending out repetitive neural stimulation associated with chronic pain. Many clients have found complete relief from their chronic pain thanks to sound therapy, including those with old injuries and phantom pain from amputation. Additionally, sound therapy enhances sleep quality and reduces stress, which at the very least, makes dealing with a condition like chronic pain more tolerable.

A more recent form of sound therapy called vibroacoustic therapy employs audible sound vibrations to lessen symptoms, promote relaxation, and reduce stress. This technology was developed in Norway by Olav Skille in response to the realization that external vibrations can directly affect specific body functions. The effectiveness of vibroacoustic therapy has been extensively studied.

Lower-frequency brain waves can trigger the release of nitric oxide, which signals smooth muscles to relax, allowing blood vessels to expand improving blood flow. Some scientists contend that this release of nitric oxide alters how we perceive pain because it positively impacts how pain is managed and transmitted.

Addiction

Stress and anxiety are fundamental elements that obstruct recovery from substance abuse. By implementing specific sound therapy concepts, vibration, resonance, and rhythm are carefully administered to reduce stress and promote healthy cellular changes.

In addition to managing the addiction's physical effects, clients can address its emotional and mental impacts by combining sound, rhythm, and vibration with other conventional or alternative therapies, such as individual or group sessions, yoga, brain mapping, exercise, or acupuncture.

In most cases, addiction also results in the emergence of a co-occurring disorder (or vice versa), and simply getting clean from the substance is insufficient for a complete and sustained recovery. Clients must also treat the underlying causes of their destructive behavior above and beyond merely focusing on the associated physical and emotional symptoms. By addressing addiction at the brain wave level with sound therapy, medical professionals can help clients enter meditative states more readily and confront their issues.

Music and meditation tracks can be a potent ally in the quest for finding purpose and meaning in life when used in conjunction with other therapeutic modalities. Through the use of music or other sound sources, sound therapy can help people rediscover their emotional core and address specific underlying issues that are present. An additional benefit of sound therapy is that it can lessen boredom and loneliness, which are two significant contributors associated with relapse.

Aging

Sound therapy is an effective, non-invasive method to support healthy aging. It promotes a deep relaxation state conducive to healing. Numerous research sources acknowledge sound therapy as a powerful method of coping with ongoing stress, which slows the aging process, strengthens the immune system and lifts a person's spirit. Throughout the aging process, seniors can benefit from sound therapy's ability to increase focus and memory, lessen pain, boost healthy hormones that fight stress and sleep deprivation, reduce anxiety and depression, and increase brain activity, improving emotional and mental clarity.

Appetite and Digestion

Another line of research reveals that while cooking sounds like sizzling bacon or popping corn may make your mouth water, sounds like chewing, chomping, and crunching food are more likely to turn you off. Studies have previously listed taste, texture, meal size, and food choice as sensory cues that affect satiety, or the sense of having consumed an adequate quantity of food. Presently, there is an expanding knowledge base about the factors that influence people's preferences toward specific types and quantities of food.

Elaborating on this line of study, more recent research developments encourage people to imagine the sounds of eating, even utilizing advertisements to assist in reducing excessive consumption. In other words, people may instinctively eat less when they are more conscious of the sound their food makes while they are eating. This has been referred to as the "Crunch Effect."

Consumers and researchers generally ignore the impact of the sound of food, despite it being a significant sensory cue in the eating experience. However, the hypothesis is that food consumption would decrease with an increased awareness of the distinct sounds produced while eating. When the sound of consumption is muffled, as when eating while watching television, one of the vital senses connected to food is eliminated. Thus, the inverse may be actualized as an increase in food consumption. This being said, it may prove beneficial to pay attention to the *sound* of food in addition to how it tastes and looks when actively implementing weight loss goals.

Arthritis & Rheumatism

Rheumatism and arthritis are umbrella terms for more than a hundred diseases and conditions that cause pain, swelling, stiffness, and joint inflammation. Although there isn't a curative treatment for many of them presently, techniques like ultrasound therapy can help lessen the discomfort.

Treatment for arthritic pain using ultrasound therapy is a successful, non-invasive method, during which the body's soft tissues experience intense heating, which lessens localized pain. It is also possible to combine ultrasound therapy with other forms of physical therapy, such as electrical stimulation, to increase the effectiveness of pain management.

Ultrasound therapy also comes with a lot of versatility. Practitioners can essentially treat any part of the body, from the lower back to the elbows, as a broad selection of soundhead applicators is available. Practitioners can also choose between continuous or pulsed ultrasound therapy to treat trigger point pain, deep tissue, or superficial skin concerns.

Blood Pressure

Music can reduce stress, ease recovery from cardiac procedures, help patients rebound after heart attacks or strokes, and even help lower blood pressure. A large body of research supports the powerful healing effects of sound for regulating hypertension.

Heart patients confined to bed for 30 minutes while listening to music experienced lower blood pressure, slower heart rates, and less distress than those who did not. For four weeks, older patients who listened to calming music for 25 minutes each day reduced their systolic (the top number in a blood pressure reading) and diastolic (the bottom number) pressures by 12 and 5 points, respectively. In contrast, older patients who did not listen to music experienced no improved change in blood pressure.

A recently developed sound therapy application shows promise in lowering blood pressure and easing migraine symptoms. The treatment first uses scalp sensors to measure brain activity. A series of audible tones are then generated from the collected data. In merely milliseconds, the interventional tones are transmitted back through earbuds to the brain.

It is neither a drug nor an invasive procedure. Through this treatment, the patient's systolic blood pressure decreased on average from 152 to 136 mm Hg; their diastolic pressure decreased from 97 to 81 mm Hg. Per the present medical standard, the normal blood pressure target is 120/80 mm Hg or less.

Approximately 400 people participated in a series of studies evaluating this therapy, known as high-resolution, relational, resonance-based, electro-encephalic mirroring (HIRREM; Thompson, 2016). Through the means of a neural biofeedback mechanism, this treatment aids in the realignment of the autonomic nervous system. Our internal organs are intrinsically regulated by the autonomic nervous system, which also subsequently controls vital bodily processes like respiration, digestion, and heart rate. Independent research has shown that it can help with treatment for people who struggle with stress, anxiety, depression, and insomnia.

Cancers

Medical professionals in Britain have begun employing potent ultrasound beams to eliminate harmful tissue deep within the bodies of patients with metastatic bone lesions. This procedure, known as high-intensity focused ultrasound (HIFU), may revolutionize cancer treatment because it eliminates the need for pricy and invasive surgery (Julious, 2020).

Focused ultrasound proves effective because it can target tumors with pinpoint accuracy. This technology is comparable to using a magnifying glass in the sun to form a sharp focal spot on dry tinder to start a fire. HIFU has shown promise in patients with recurrent gynecological cancers and secondary tumors in the bone and offers great promise for the future regarding other cancers.

UK researchers further found that sound wave therapy was a successful treatment for 90% of male patients with prostate cancer, devoid of any unfavorable side effects. (Chase, 2015)

Along other lines relative to cancer, circulating tumor cells (CTCs) can be successfully and quickly separated from blood using sound waves. CTCs are microscopic tumor fragments that separate and move through the bloodstream. They are incredibly informative, containing details about the genetic mutations, physical characteristics, and types of tumors. These "liquid biopsies," as the researchers dubbed them, could one day assist oncologists in diagnosing patients and developing more individualized treatment regimens without the invasiveness of a typical biopsy or screening.

Additionally, sound can support cancer patients in coping with their symptoms. Using gongs and other sound therapy methodologies allows them to feel a sense of calm and release that they typically cannot experience in any other way. The intent is to encourage the participants with a restored sense of serenity, perhaps for the first time since receiving the devastating news of a cancer diagnosis. It extends to them the impression that life still offers virtue, beauty, and worthwhileness.

Chronic Fatigue

One of the leading causes of stress and fatigue is noise. The sounds we hear immediately affect our entire system because the ear is directly connected to many other body organs through neural pathways. Sadly, the majority of the sounds we hear in our automated, urbanized way of life are low-frequency sounds through traffic, factories, home appliances, refrigerators, fluorescent lights, and even computers. These low-frequency drones deplete brain energy and lead to stress.

Sound therapy allows us an alternative where we can listen to soothing, high-frequency sounds even when we're in a crowded, noisy environment. The specific sound therapy that pertains here is through playing classical music while gradually filtering out low frequencies to leave mostly those above 8,000 Hz. This music can counteract the depleting and stressful effects of low-frequency noise when played for three hours each day as one goes about their regular routine. After six weeks to three months of following this regimen, most listeners report feeling more energized and less stressed.

Immune System

Your immune system may benefit from sound therapy as well. Sound vibrations can change how the brain functions in respect to reducing the somatic stimuli that trigger inflammation. It has been demonstrated that sound therapy can lower the production of stress hormones and cortisol, which are known to weaken the body's immune system.

Some sound therapists even assert that music can effectively lessen pain and has the power to hasten the recovery process for wounds and bone fractures. It is imperative that you seek medical guidance in the case of any major physical, mental, or emotional ailment. However, music therapy methodologies are beneficial when incorporated into a holistic health and wellness program that emphasizes general health and well-being.

Migraines

When you experience the debilitating pain from a migraine, it likely seems as though noise is the last thing you want to hear. But one of the best ways to lessen the pain brought on by one of these crippling headaches is to become more relaxed. Because soothing sounds put you at ease, developing your own sound-healing routine will help you manage your headaches. It has also been demonstrated that HIRREM sound therapy can lessen migraine symptoms.

It is already a firmly established premise throughout this book that binaural beats can be used to relieve stress and tension. By putting you in a more relaxed state of mind, these well-regulated beats make you feel more at ease and thus help lessen migraine pain when it occurs. The recommendation is to have compiled playlists containing binaural beats tracks that you have predetermined effective to manage migraine episodes quickly and easily. Binaural music is available from websites like YouTube and music streaming services like Spotify, Apple Music, and Pandora.

The theta brain wave frequency (4–8 Hz) is where most researchers advise using binaural beats for migraines. This frequency is linked to relaxation and meditation. Binaural beat proponents recommend turning down the lights, getting comfortable, and listening for at least 30 minutes to ensure your brain state synchronizes with the rhythm and harmony of the healing beats.

Sinuses—Flu, Colds, Bronchitis

A doctor who practices treating the ears, nose, and throat is known as an ENT specialist. The combination of these three body systems signifies a close interconnectedness in the medical realm, where specialization is the norm. There is no doubt that breathing involves the nose and throat. And sound therapy has an effect on these respiratory systems as well.

Sound therapy's ability to help with chronic sinus and ear blockage conditions is one of its unexpected but very real advantages. The eustachian tube muscles, closely interconnected with the middle ear muscles, frequently function suboptimally, resulting in conditions ranging from pressure in the ears to a chronically blocked ear.

Listeners claiming to suffer from chronic sinus problems have discovered that using associated sound healing techniques lessens their discomfort and frequency of attacks. There are two distinct ways to release pressure in the eustachian tubes and sinus cavities: allowing the fluid to drain, often through the placement of tubes, and decreasing buildup in the sinus cavities. The act of normal respiration is undoubtedly easier when the sinuses are unblocked. Therefore, proper implementation of sound therapy has the potential to make it easier for us to breathe, regardless of whether sinus function, emotional stress, or a stifled autonomic nervous system are affecting our breathing.

Skin

Skin is irrefutably the largest organ in your body. It prevents your internal viscera from contact with the outside environment, shielding it from germs and viruses that can infect you. It also aids body temperature regulation and allows you to sense environmental factors like temperature and humidity. Skin conditions that irritate, clog, or inflame can cause symptoms such as itching, burning, swelling, and redness.

Researchers have discovered a statistically significant improvement in the rate of healing when a slowly healing wound is exposed to low-frequency ultrasound. More research is being conducted to define this phenomenon contained within the science of sound. One possible explanation is that ultrasound encourages the development of new cells.

To expand on some additional cases, research is currently in progress offering that music therapy may offer physical and emotional relief for people with eczema. The physical aspect may require a largely technical explanation. However, emotionally, there is certainly no harm in incorporating music into your daily routine if you discover that it diverts attention from itching and scratching, lowering frustration thus making dealing with the present distresses more bearable.

The 741 Hz frequency is especially useful for clearing your cells of toxins and electromagnetic radiation. This frequency also can aid in ridding your cells of bacterial, viral, and fungal infections. Since your integumentary system – the scientific terminology for the skin system – is the front-line defense for many of these invaders, lending added support only makes sense in regard to maintaining general health and wellness.

Strong rife frequency (low electromagnetic energy waves) aids in treating a wide range of skin-related conditions and illnesses, including eczema, acne, allergies, and pimples.

Sleep

Although sound therapy revitalizes the brain for activity during the day, it also can be applied as a calming effect that makes it possible for the listener to drift off to sleep without difficulty. Stress significantly contributes to insomnia, so we naturally sleep better when sound therapy lowers stress levels. Sleeplessness is primarily brought on by uncontrolled cortical steroid overproduction. Even though the brain is exhausted from constant stress, it is unable to protect itself from the stimuli triggering it. The brain requires a calm, relaxed condition in order to enter the sleep state.

Sound therapy can assist with quieting the mental chatter so that it can shift into the slower rhythms that encourage sleep. Sound therapy helps us find the cranial 'off' button so that our mental energy can be recharged.

Counterintuitively, it is helpful for sleep to give the mind something to do. It may seem contradictory, but keeping specific brain regions occupied can lessen the busy, circling thoughts that keep us awake. The brain is actively engaged during sound therapy without being distressed or agitated, allowing the mind to relax. This aids in preventing or reducing negatively charged emotional states and lowering the risk of developing depression.

A recent survey found that between 70% and 80% of people who use sound therapy as a sleep aid report that it has helped them sleep better (Sleep, Insomnia, and Sound Therapy, 2017). Through the stimulation of the brain and nervous system, sound can induce an active serenity that encourages deep sleep. Additionally, anxiety-related insomnia usually goes away. When the ear is exposed to high-frequency sounds, which mimic the experience of pre-birth, early emotional apprehensions can be more easily overcome. Delta brain wave music, which ranges in frequency from 0.5 to 4 Hz, is known to aid in sleep quality and quantity by helping people drift off more quickly with fewer awakenings. Through this use of sound therapy, many people with insomnia have noticed immediate and significantly improved sleep.

Weight Gain or Loss

Sound and music are frequently used to create a calming environment for listeners in sound baths. A stress-eating sound bath combines the calming effects of sound and music with chimes, steel tongue drums, crystal (or Tibetan) singing bowls, or other instruments designed to calm listeners while altering motivations.

Some of the secrets are hidden in specific frequencies, like the solfeggio scale and 432 Hz. Research has demonstrated that these particular frequencies can be both calming and healing. When used to treat emotional eating, stress eating, or food addiction, the intention is to use sound to encourage the listener to focus on an alternate source of release than eating when they are anxious or upset.

Focusing on the sound during a sound bath slows the listener's brain waves, which relaxes them. In some cases, the practitioner will point out circumstances that might have led the listener to give in to food cravings and help them visualize shifting their attention and behavior. By doing this, the listener is given the tools necessary to avoid giving in to food cravings the next time they are confronted with a stressful situation.

Music has a significant impact on workouts, which means that it indirectly affects metabolic rates. Music can facilitate increasing serotonin levels and lowering cortisol levels, improving mood and energy levels. Higher serotonin levels are correlated with better metabolic rates. You can lose weight more quickly if you approach your weight loss efforts in a relaxed state of mind. A tense and demanding mind can lead to weight gain, whereas music calms the senses and promotes weight loss.

Note: While music therapy is beneficial for treating all these aspects of well-being, if you are experiencing severe or persistent symptoms of any sort, including those below, it is crucial that you seek external medical help.

- very high or persistent fever
- flashes of light or bright spots in your vision
- sudden breathing difficulties
- early satiety, which might be accompanied by nausea, vomiting, bloating, or weight loss.
- sudden and unexplained changes in bowel habits, such as bloody, black, or tarry stools, ongoing diarrhea or constipation, or unexplained urges to urinate.
- loss of weight without cause (if you are not obese and have inadvertently lost more than 10 pounds or 5% of your body weight in the last six to twelve months.)
- changes in personality or mental status such as altered thinking, trouble focusing, maintaining consciousness, or attention shifts.

THE FREQUENCIES OF THE HUMAN ANATOMY

Vibrational stimulus-related concerns are now a commonplace occurrence in people's daily lives. These stimuli can harm people's health and interfere with their daily activities. Numerous factors contribute to these issues, including the expansion of air traffic and the number of heavy vehicles that act as unwelcome sources of noise and vibration in urban areas.

The human body can be viewed as a multi-degree-of-freedom complex system. Our body's organs each have a unique range of resonance frequencies. Understanding these frequencies allows us to choose the methods and tools to support any health-related challenge we encounter.

Organs	Resonance Frequencies (Hz)
Head	20 to 40
Spinal column	8
Chest wall	60
Abdominal	4 to 8
Shoulders	4 to 8
Lungs	4 to 8
Hands and arms	20 to 70
Ocular globe	60 to 90
Maxilla	100 to 200

(Duarte & de Brito Pereira, 2006)

Music therapy and sound healing support more than just our physical needs. They also work wonders for our mental and emotional needs.

6

SOUND HEALING FOR THE MIND AND HEART

Sound and Resonance is the common denominator of religions & creation; it connects us and leads us towards higher Consciousness.

— MICHAEL TELLINGER

SOUND HEALING FOR MENTAL AND EMOTIONAL WELL-BEING

It is always advisable to seek the assistance of a therapist or counselor when dealing with significant mental or emotional concerns because they can provide you with the tools needed to better manage any symptoms you may be experiencing. In some cases, taking medications prescribed by a psychiatrist or medical professional can offer restorative treatment that can assist the brain in healing.

Music therapy and sound therapy are very effective when it comes to identifying and controlling mental and emotional states. Music therapy can ease tension and encourage rest. It has been demonstrated in the clinical setting to be more successful than prescription medications at lowering anxiety levels prior to surgery. Because of its capacity to alter brain chemistry, music therapy is also an effective countermeasure for various mental health issues, including depression. Sound therapy aims to use calming sounds to create harmony and balance. Implementing the benefits of sound therapy range from simply listening to music, nature sounds, or chanting to monitored administeration by a qualified professional.

Cognitive Health

The application of music in cognitive therapy has advanced quickly as brain imaging techniques have revealed the brain's plasticity — its capacity to evolve and remap synaptic connections in response to circumstantial exposure — and have identified the neural networks that music activates. With this expanding scope of knowledge, medical professionals and academics are turning to music to help injured brains recover. As a result of shared neural circuits between music and motor control, studies have demonstrated that music can improve fine-motion management in patients experiencing strokes or Parkinson's disease. It is argued that these practices should be incorporated into rehabilitative care because research has shown that neurologic music therapy can benefit patients exhibiting difficulties speaking or thinking clearly.

In Alzheimer's care facilities, it is common to observe patients, who cannot recall their first names, singing upbeat old songs like "Cheek to Cheek" and other familiar tunes with surprising vigor. Similarly, the ability of certain stroke patients with dysphasia (difficulty speaking) to sing along to their favorite songs, not demonstrating any speech deficiencies, has long been noted by clinicians.

People with Parkinson's disease, a neurodegenerative disorder that affects movement and most often leads to difficulties walking, have demonstrated notable improvements in their mobility when they synchronize their footsteps with a musical rhythm or tempo. In essence, when these patients align the timing of their steps to the beat of a song, they can walk better and with greater ease.

The most significant part of our musical knowledge and many of its representations, such as structure and character, come from natural exposure. Babies learn music long before birth, memorizing it so well that after birth, without hearing it again in the interim, they can recognize it a year or more later. At the other end of life, music is still accessible even when linguistic capabilities diminish. In addition to inspiring the desire to speak, smile, and sing, it also brings back memories and occasions associated with the music. This is especially notable for people with advanced Alzheimer's disease.

While the right brain handles perceptive analysis – i.e., recognition of a melody – the left brain's regions associated with musical memory and language allow us to name a musical work specifically. This particular arrangement makes music memory superior to verbal memory. When a patient exhibits a left-brain injury (affecting language), the corresponding right-brain regions do not typically compensate for this deficit. The majority of the time, though, the patient can still enjoy listening to music, even memorizing songs, though perhaps not being able to name them.

Numerous studies demonstrate that, in the case of brain lesions, stimulating the brain's music-processing zone positively impacts cognitive abilities (attention, memory, and language processing) and encourages brain plasticity. All ages, including the elderly, who start listening to music later in life, can benefit from the positive effects on the brain's general cognitive functioning. Studies on stroke patients have revealed that these individuals not only enjoy listening to music that evokes memories, but they further involuntarily start humming these tunes. This response aids in the brain's functional reorganization necessary for recovering linguistic ability.

Fear Management: Anxiety, Stress, Panic Attacks

Music has a powerful impact on both the body and emotions. Music with a faster tempo often enhances your mood and focus. Listening to upbeat music inspires you to feel more positive and relaxed about life. Slower music can tame your thoughts and unwind your physical tensions while relieving other stress points, overall having a welcome calming effect. Music has the power to help people relax and regulate their anxiety.

These individualized musical experiences are supported by research. Listening to music playing at 60 beats per minute or higher has been verified to synchronize the mental state with the 8 to 14 Hz alpha brain waves, the state at which we are simultaneously at ease and cognitive. Sleep requires the delta brain wave state of 5 Hz. To attain entering this state may require at least 45 minutes of listening to relaxing music in a comfortable environment. Increased studies on the effects of sound and music on human behavior have purported that listening to music alters brain function to the same degree as medication. These studies emphasize implementing sound and music as stress-reduction tools, noting their effectiveness for anyone with the capacity to listen.

Surprisingly for some, it seems that Native American, Celtic, and Eastern Indian stringed instruments, drums, and flutes are the most effective at calming the mind, even when played at moderate volumes. Rain, thunder, and other sounds found in nature can also be soothing, especially when combined with various types of music like light jazz, classical (most typically "largo" movements), and easy listening.

The point that we often lack the vital information of adequately knowing a song's average tempo in beats per minute makes it challenging to choose the optimal music for relaxation. However, a significant part of the solution lies within oneself. To be effective, the music must first be personally enjoyable before it can transform you into a relaxed state. The recommendation is to start by listening to music readily available to you, whether from your personal collection or any of numerous online sources. The simple reality is that some songs will help you relax while others will not. It will actually increase tension if you force yourself to listen to "calming" music that irritates you. When that happens, search for alternatives online or ask guidance from a professional music therapist for additional recommendations. A large part of this process is developing effective playlists and sources personalized to your individual emotive response. Be especially cognitive of the fact that clearing your mind does not necessarily result in falling asleep; it as often means that your body and mind being at ease allows you to perform various tasks at your fullest potential.

Anger Management

Anger has a unique impact on each individual and can manifest in any number of ways. These consist of harboring resentments intending to exact revenge, violent outbursts, or a persistent internalized feeling of rage. This emotion can harm friendships, family, and work relationships when it is unchecked or expressed unduly or inappropriately. In reality, a person's physical health can be affected by anger because it significantly elevates blood pressure, increasing the risk of heart disease and other severe physiological and psychological conditions.

The overall intent of using music therapy with clients who need anger management is to help them better regulate their anger. However, numerous smaller objectives support the accomplishment of the main goal, whether it be identifying the memories or experiences that cause persisting resentment or creating a set of coping mechanisms. These objectives assist clients in determining the causes of their outbursts of uncontrollable rage and aid them in formulating healthier responses to those occasions. Additional goals are to become more aware of unchecked negative emotions and learn relaxation techniques.

One of the music therapy interventions used in prisons is lyrical analysis. Lyrical analysis offers clients opportunity to engage with and analyze the lyrics of well-known songs. Clients can then evaluate their own thought processes and emotions in light of the lyrics' expression and meaning. This enables them to connect with their feelings.

Performance is yet another frequent intervention strategy. Clients move to physically express their emotions, mimic everyday tasks, and think about how they use space by changing their body language and exercising verbal control.

Clients can also write their own song lyrics while occasionally performing them. They can use this as a journal-type alternative to express and evaluate their thoughts and feelings. Through this avenue of articulation coupled with performance, clients can express their thoughts and feelings in a healthy and productive way.

Self-Worth

The power of vibrational sound is the embodiment of sound healing. Our physical bodies and minds are fed by the frequencies of specific sounds, which enable us to heal internally. The frequency of 528 Hz helps to balance and tune the Solar Plexus Chakra or energy system, which supports self-assurance and self-esteem. This includes soothing sleep music based on the 528 Hz solfeggio frequency, also referred to as the Love Frequency, the Miracle Tone, or the Frequency of Transformation. This frequency promotes change and reformation while encouraging positive vibes.

Attending a sound therapy session can help you foster a positive outlook and increase your self-confidence. By following a carefully planned sound therapy session, you can accomplish several life tasks previously regarded as daunting or unachievable. It is strongly recommended to search out reputable facilities that offer the best sound therapy experience to bolster your self-esteem.

Negative Thinking

Science and common sense have proven that listening to music you enjoy makes you happier. However, since we can see it for ourselves in our daily lives, we hardly need the scientific proof for it. Your favorite music every day demonstrates its ability to lessen your response to stressful situations. This is effective, encompassing a broad scope of life, including anything from reducing the ill effect of a bad smell to making physically taxing work less of a chore.

Another way that music can help cope with negativity is by enabling a person to better manage their emotions. The capacity to better manage these emotions enhances your ability to respond to, be sustained through, and process unfavorable circumstances. Embracing this understanding and all that it implies empowers you that when you encounter negative emotions, their effect will be for a shorter period of time and that those emotions will not exercise as much control over you while they are present.

To assist in attaining this status, sound baths are a powerful tool for deeply reaching and altering the subconscious mind. These sessions can be used as a means of relaxation and personal growth. We can use this tool to purge undesirable habits or thought patterns. It can serve as the foundation for renewed mental tendencies, routines, and paths in life.

Depression

Although it is commonly known that an imbalance in brain chemistry causes depression, the precise interactions of this chemistry are very complex and are still not fully understood. We know it involves how the brain produces and utilizes certain neurochemicals, such as serotonin and dopamine. These neurotransmitters, or brain chemicals, influence our feelings of joy and elation.

The good news is that because the body has a natural capacity to heal itself, it can do so if the proper environment and elements support the process. Although chemicals play a crucial role in this operation, there is mounting evidence that activating our sensory systems has a profound influence on the chemicals that our brain produces and uses. And for our purposes, sound can serve well as that stimulus.

Sound therapy has demonstrated that it can help depressed individuals by stimulating the brain via aural channels of an affected person with massive amounts of high-frequency sounds. Since these vibrations have a high energy level, they energize the listener. Sound therapy additionally triggers the brain to naturally produce neurotransmitters activating positive emotions. Clients of sound therapy frequently express more significant levels of well-being, joy, and reduction or resolution of depression symptoms.

Furthermore, research shows that a key factor in the therapeutic effect against depression is the targeted stimulation of the left brain. Accompanying studies on the impact of meditation being practiced regularly indicates activation for parts of the left forebrain that promote these feelings of joy and peace. Similar results have been seen when the left brain is directly stimulated by sound therapy through an increase in high-frequency sound input to the right ear.

With alpha, delta, or theta music, binaural beats can also promote a deeply relaxed state, an improved mood, a healthier sleep cycle, increased focus, and reduced anxiety, all of which contribute to reducing depression symptoms.

BRAIN WAVES AND THEIR EFFECTS

The previous chapters have covered how various external stimuli, including auditory stimulation, can change brain wave patterns. Researchers continue to debate the precise frequency thresholds, but those listed below are typically accurate within a few hertz.

While this is a practical method of categorization, some academics also point out that it disregards the extraordinarily intricate and largely unrecognized interrelationships that exist between frequencies. The field of brain wave research is still very much a work in progress.

Similar to how each of our body's organs has a unique resonance frequency, each type of brain wave has an associated function and resonating frequency. The more knowledge we acquire about which brain waves are associated with which mental and emotional states and what frequencies can elicit those states, the more adept and proactive we can be in choosing the proper sound-healing equipment and associated sonic implementations.

Brain Wave	Frequency (Hz)	Benefits and Functions
Gamma	32–100	The ability to learn, focus, and exercise restraint
Beta	12–38	Elevated levels of energy, concentration, alertness, and clarity of thought
Alpha	8–12	Help with memory, mild anxiety, tension headaches, and states of creative flow
Theta	3.5–7.5	Improved memory consolidation, intuition, deep relaxation, and emotional processing
Delta	0.5–4	Support healing, deep sleep, and immune and inflammatory system function.

Sound has the power to heal in a multitude of ways, including those that affect our mental, emotional, and physical health. But it doesn't end there. There is also the matter of our spiritual health. The emergence of our spiritual self can be significantly influenced by sound.

7

SOUND HEALING FOR THE SOUL

Take a music bath once or twice a week for a few seasons, and you will find that it is to the soul what the water bath is to the body.

— OLIVER WENDELL HOLMES

SOUND IN OUR SPIRITUAL JOURNEY

Matter, energy, sound, and form are all intertwined. Consider the example of water to put this in perspective. In his book The Hidden Messages in Water, Masaru Emoto explains how water exposed to human motivation that is loving, kind, and compassionate creates physically pleasing molecular manifestations, whereas water exposed to influences that are fearful and discordant creates disconnected, deformed, and unpleasant molecular formations. He accomplished this using high-speed photography and magnetic resonance analysis technology (Emoto, 2004, as cited in Durkin, 2017).

Sound has the power to invoke spiritual experiences. Since the dawn of time, sound and music have been used by cultures throughout the world to aid in spiritual healing, harmony, and awakening.

Many individuals believe that spiritual healing consists merely of purging ourselves of unhelpful feelings, severe emotional problems, and unreliable belief systems in order to better resonate with love and light. Some also view it from a psychological angle, arguing that we must achieve mental clarity to prevent our thoughts from constantly leading us down stressful, anxiety-provoking paths that are roller coasters and dead-end traps that result in recursive states of stress and anxiety. We've already discussed how sound can be therapeutic for these psychological and emotional problems.

But sound possesses virtue able to go well beyond that, drawing us into harmony and establishing a direct line of communication with spirit, soul, and source. When we forge a close bond with our soul and learn to hear it speak instead of our ego and personality, we often receive guidance on how to live our lives more fulfilled.

Furthermore, it is logical to assume that the root frequency upon which our entire body is based must exist at every level. Everything in the universe resonates with a fundamental note, just as every sound has a rudimentary frequency, every song has a home key, etc. Research conducted in hospitals has demonstrated that when you resonate with this core root frequency, your entire system becomes harmonious.

Music has always been a conduit between substance and spirit — an ethereal influence that unites us through the language of the heart — from the Amazonian medicine songs to euphoric Gospel hymns and Gregorian chants. Sound and music can help connect with the higher energies of what many refer to as Spirit, Source, or God. Music transports us to a different realm when we truly listen to it. Perhaps this explains why sound has been used as a form of prayer by virtually every culture and civilization.

Even if you already have a way to communicate with Spirit, the right music and sounds can fortify it. While specific frequencies may inspire it, it happens more frequently when specific sounds (resonances) or musical intervals and rhythms are used in a song. You can also perform this energetically while establishing your inspiration. When all levels of frequency, resonance, music, and energy are working together, entire worlds of unimaginable healing power and consciousness levels that we have never previously considered can open before us.

Forgetting about ourselves through singing or listening is what prayer is all about. We release a call from the inner depths out of our thirst for freedom. Music, which awakens the soul's yearning, serves as this reminder.

Religious Practices

Numerous religious traditions share a connection between music and spirituality. Music has always been a part of religious ceremonies and worship since the beginning of time, as shown by customs from various cultures and geographical areas.

The musical traditions that accompany each religion serve as a symbol for the various religiously inspired musical practices. Hindu meditative music, for instance, employs bronze instruments from Indonesia. In contrast, rock band music, Russian Orthodox choir, and Gregorian chants are all included in contemporary Christian music. There are diverse musical practices from various parts of the world, even within the same religious traditions. These sacred music traditions contain a variety of expressive forms, such as melodic, repetitive vocalizations known as chants; piercing, passionate, and emotionally charged groans, shouts, and hums; synchronized and rhythmic hand claps and foot stomps; and lengthy hymns and instrumental compositions.

Throughout history, people have used instrumental music, sung prayers, and mystical chants to express their moral, political, social, and economic aspirations, as well as to communicate with the divine and to bring together diverse religious communities. Calling upon the spirits is primarily accomplished through sacred sounds in many traditions. Many cultures hold the belief that making certain sounds creates a connection with all the elements of the universe. According to some religious and philosophical traditions, sound and music vibrations can heal the body, mind, and spirit. One of the most potent and inspiring ways for all peoples and cultures to acknowledge the nature of the Supreme in their lives is through the ability to incorporate the joys, sorrows, and humility that define religious and spiritual beliefs into oral poetry, chants, songs, and instrumental music.

Religious music also affects a person's psychological state by evoking a spectrum of feelings and thought processes. Some sacred music, such as the gospel genre, conveys a message of optimism and hope. It implies that the more often one listens to spiritual music, the less fear one has of dying. Those given to its influence often seem happier with their lives and feel better about themselves.

Religious music holds the values of fostering community and encouraging participation. When people praise and give thanks to a higher power together, a strong sense of unified solidarity permeates the group's actions and attitudes. When religious music is performed, audiences in many religious communities start to physically respond to the music by swaying back and forth. With time, this engagement gets stronger. As the swaying grows more synchronized and coordinated, even those who remain still eventually start to sway along. A group's unity can be fostered through music while promoting peace in the sacred, reverent setting.

Shamanic Sound Journeys

In nearly every setting where shamanism is practiced, music or sound is an essential part of the ritual. Using sound as a form of energetic mechanism, it aligns our existential vibration to deliberate harmonic frequencies by interacting with our human energy field.

When it comes to shamanic practices, sound healing pays homage to the first iterations of traditional shamanism that used sound as a portal to the spirit realms. The method and mentality of shamanic sound healing involve using sound in rituals and ceremonies to help information and healing energy flow from the divine spiritual realms to Earth. When one invites the wisdom and power of compassionate aiding spirits to work with them while making sound, the results have been noted as astoundingly magnified, far-reaching, and unfathomable in the most remarkable ways. This is particularly true when considering one's resolve to hold ceremonies in conjunction with each shamanic transmission.

Shamanic sound healing is an ethereal, artistic, liberating experience. Whether you need healing, want to motivationally integrate sound and spirit into your personal or professional life, or desire to incorporate sound into shamanic healing rituals or other energy medicine practices, you can become an agent of shamanic sound healing.

Shamanic sound healing, also known as a shamanic sound bath, uses musical instruments like gongs, tuning forks, and Tibetan singing bowls to bathe or flood a ceremony participant's energetic space with resonant vibrations that are intended to relieve stress, anxiety, and energy blockages. This process aims to help participants find a greater sense of peace and purpose in life.

Along with the shamanic drum, which is the primary instrument used by shamanistic healers, they use their voices and the aforementioned instruments. A shamanic drum is played in steady harmonic rhythms that are either channeled or intentionally maintained. These rhythms are typically fast (4–7 beats per second) and constant. The sound of this drum can be compared to the heartbeat, which is regarded as the universally calming sound of life.

The ultimate goal of shamanic sound healing is to surround the client's body and aura in healing vibrations so that the chakras can attain balance. This is always performed with the intention of improving the client's overall sense of well-being beyond simply their physical and emotional health.

Chakras

Another noted source of sound healing uses particular frequencies that resonate throughout the body to balance the chakras. It works by harmonizing with each chakra's specific sound frequency. When your chakras are balanced, your entire being — body, mind, and spirit — is vibrant and healthy.

Chakras are energy nodes in your body that are situated along your spine. Your chakras' energy pathways, or nadis, are what feed them life energy. They act as your body's equivalent of an energy network. There are 72,000 nadis, which are connected at seven major centers. These seven primary energy centers are known as the root chakra, sacral chakra, solar plexus chakra, heart chakra, throat chakra, third eye chakra, and crown chakra.

The chakra system is one of the elements of your energy body. The vibrational frequency of your energy body serves as the blueprint for your life. Because ancient Indian cultures were aware of how the body's energy flows, they developed methods for working with these energies.

Our energy body is disturbed by trauma, fears, and insecurities brought on by life experiences. When this occurs, our prana, or life force, doesn't flow easily; it gets restricted in some places, causing insufficient energy. Your chakras become unbalanced, making you more susceptible to both physical and mental illnesses. Sound has the power to harmonize your chakras.

Sound healing employs specific sound frequencies to harmonize a person's mind and body. You can heal your chakras with a plethora of different sound-producing devices. Tibetan singing bowls, gongs, and tuning forks are the most traditional and well-preferred tools for chakra healing. A more contemporary variation is the use of crystal singing bowls and pyramids. Every chakra vibrates at a particular frequency. Applying that frequency to your body will cause your chakra to realign, giving you the energy you need to be vibrant and healthy.

Chakra	Color	Frequency (Hz)	Musical Note
Root	Red	432	C
Sacral	Orange or Vermillion	480	D
Solar Plexus	Yellow	528	E
Heart	Green	594	F
Throat	Blue	672	G
Third Eye	Blue or Purple	720	A
Crown	Violet	768	B

Mantras, Affirmations, and Visualizations

According to ancient texts, the 108 sound frequencies produced by the motion of celestial bodies in different constellations can be heard throughout the universe. Every sound has a specific frequency, so whenever you repeat a mantra, you directly and unavoidably combine these 108 frequencies. Suppose you've chanted the mantra enough and produced sufficient sound frequency; in this case, the frequencies you create will eventually align with those in the cosmos. This connection will heal and bring harmony to your mind, body, and environment.

Use a mantra, for instance, with the intent to manifest wealth, better interpersonal relationships, or enhance your health and well-being. In addition, a mantra targeted explicitly to a particular motivation can help you connect to the frequency of desire to manifest positive changes in your life. In this way, a mantra serves as a tool for both connecting with the universe and bringing your awareness back to your inner self.

Many people have recited specific mantras millions of times. As a result, those mantras become extremely powerfully charged with frequency energy. A mentor, guru, or master typically provides a charged mantra for the purpose of spiritual development. Someone who has already completed this mantra and attained its power can initiate another individual into it. In this case, a very potent, powerful mantra of quality may be transferred.

Everyone is born with between six and ten different sound frequencies. One can recognize these sound frequencies individually and then practice them repeatedly for overall well-being, harmony, and healing. They can be applied in a targeted manner to achieve specific goals.

Chanting amplifies this effect because it causes vibrations inside and outside your body, keeping you thoroughly present with the sound. When you repeat a mantra to yourself, you, the mantra, and the purpose for which you are repeating it all meld into one.

Crystal Use

Crystal sound therapy is a centuries-old technique where sound healers use quartz crystal singing bowls to create various sound frequencies to re-establish harmony and balance in the body. Crystal sound healing is regarded as a holistic healing method because it influences the mind, body, emotions, and spirit. It slows down brain waves, which promotes deep relaxation and helps the body heal itself naturally.

The sound vibrations produced by crystal bowls and other comparable musical instruments are deeply relaxing, clear the chakras of outdated energies, and promote balance and lightness.

Quartz crystals emit electromagnetic energy. They store vibrationally charged light and knowledge. Lightworkers have used them for centuries to connect to higher states of power and thought.

Pure quartz crystals are now used to make singing bowls. The purpose of the bowls is to restore a harmonious vibration to any parts of the energy body that may be out of balance. Thanks to modern technology, we can now create crystal bowls of the highest quality. Such crystal quality being available increases the power of their frequencies and their effectiveness as a result.

Therapists and healers can determine vibrational imbalance by striking each bowl and moving it along the body. An imbalance is recognized when the tone of the bowl changes as it passes over the body. With the help of the sounds produced by the crystal singing bowls, the practitioner can then replace the conflicting vibration with the correct one. When the physical body is vibrating at the proper frequency, symptoms of concern should resolve, and the energetic and mental bodies restored can then vibrate appropriately. Optimal health is the ultimate objective.

This distinctive method of healing and wellness, when combined with the age-old principles of sound healing, can be compelling.

Sacred Geometry

The fact that sound represents sacred geometry has largely been kept secret from most civilizations for many years. Chinese, Indians, Tibetans, ancient Muslims, Pythagoreans, Egyptians, and members of the Islamic world were all notable proponents of this universal knowledge. Pythagoras was the first to popularize the notion that the universe is a 'celestial' or 'divine' monochord of vibratory energy from which everything resonated into existence. He was researching musical geometry, intending to comprehend cosmic laws. In nature, from plants to galaxies, golden spirals surround us and our bodies; all of nature is built using the golden ratio. Sound and music are no exception, though the geometrical elements are somewhat more abstract and sometimes elusive. Many notable pieces demonstrate characteristics consistent with the mathematical theory of the golden ratio. With sounds that we perceive as "lovely" or "beautiful," the correlation is more prominent. And certainly, contemporary artists specifically compose with this premise in mind. Yet, overall, undeniably, life consists of sacred geometry and harmony.

Yet rarely is this pertinent information imparted. It has the potential to liberate our minds by bringing to light how perfect we truly are forged. Suppose we are unaware of and do not value the perfection of our minds and bodies; how can we hope to create a harmonious and ideal inner or outer world?

By a miracle of nature, we develop from a pair of single cells into an embryo, a child, and ultimately an adult. On a cellular level, when happiness and harmony are present, the cells' corresponding vibrations cause them to arrange themselves into real mandalas of connections. In contrast, when stress is present, tensions emerge that create discord and chaos, which are then followed by disease and imbalance.

A sound that emanates sacred geometry can help us re-establish our connection to inner harmony and our own sacred geometry. We have access to many instruments that we can use or conjoin to create such balance. The singing bowl is the most widely used device that emits geometrically sacred vibrations. You can now find crystal and Himalayan singing bowls in almost every yoga studio and spa. Furthermore, they have also begun to play their role in hospitals, hospices, charity organizations that support women, children, and the elderly even military organizations that deal with post-traumatic stress syndrome patients.

Existing scientific institutions can analyze the frequencies in your voice to assess your health. Internal organs can recover their health as a result of being exposed to the proper frequencies. Following the diagnosis, a regimen for tuning into the beneficial frequencies can be established to restore those missing, promoting healing of the body.

Elaborating on one such instance, NASA conducted an experiment because astronauts' bone densities were declining due to a lack of gravity in space. Spacemen were instructed to tune into the "frequency of the bones," which sent the proper signals to the brain. Upon returning to Earth, their bones were in good functional order (Lhamo, 2019).

There is sound all around us, and it impacts essentially everything we do. One needs the proper context and environment for sound to be used purposefully. Many populations have been socialized to feel as though they lack their own voice and thus are reluctant to express it. What if, on the contrary, you were told that your voice is your distinct blueprint? Knowing this, would you be inspired to sing aloud more, pay closer attention to your voice, and listen to music that brings you peace, harmony, and health? We should use these advantages with greater awareness and intent.

8

SOUND IN REAL-TIME

The music is all around us, all you have to do is listen.

— AUGUST RUSH

Knowing the impactful influence of sound can make you more conscious of how you use it in your home, place of employment, and other settings. When you begin to take charge of the sounds surrounding you, you will start considering what sounds to include and exclude, what sounds need to be reduced or enhanced, and what significance you want the sound to have on you as well as other people who are sharing your sonic environment.

THE INFLUENCE OF SOUND SETTINGS ON MOOD AND BEHAVIOR

In all of our daily activities, sound surrounds and supports us. It also plays a vital role in our ability to survive by putting us in touch with the things around us, including but not limited to the ambiance, space, nature, objects, and human activity. We use the sounds we hear for bilateral communication, whether through listening to or expressing auditory words, sighs, expressive and emphatic tones, or any other behavioral sound cues. We are alerted or warned using the signaling character of sound. We have cell phones that ring when we receive calls or messages and trains that employ sound to alert people in the vicinity that they are approaching crossings. The same is true for any car, truck, or vehicle whose drivers use their horns to warn or attract other people's attention. Without sound, it would be impossible to conduct phone conversations that are such an extensive part of today's society.

All these sounds evoke different emotions and sensations, even triggering memories of events we associate with them. However, most sound cues are not intentionally or conscientiously produced; they just happen. Yet, with a heightened awareness of your sonic environment, you can often increase control over the soundscape, making it more suitable for certain activities, enhancing desirable moods, and making vital sound cues more effective.

Social Events

We are impacted by sound in four distinct and diverse ways: physically, psychologically, cognitively, and behaviorally.

Physical

A startling sound compels us to physically react by making our heart race, causing us to flinch or jump or want to adopt a defensive pose or sprint away. On the other hand, a comforting sound, like the sound of the ocean, may cause us to stop, extend our arms, and lift our head to heighten our listening so we can take in the calming, steadying influence of the sound which inspires us to feel open and receptive.

Psychological

We can all attest to the uplifting power of music. A punchy beat will energize and motivate us while working out. Or well-directed, fabricated ambient sounds might scare us just a little, as when the creepy music cues from a horror film commence. Music can even make us want to cry or be deeply emotionally inspired, as when listening to most songs by Adele.

Cognitive

How often have you admonished your child, your cat, or your dog to stop doing whatever they were involved in from an adjoining room? You didn't need to witness the actions taking place with your eyes to understand what was transpiring. The audio cues were sufficient to alert you to respond accordingly.

There are limits to how much auditory information our brains can process simultaneously. When it comes to sensory input from our eyes and ears, they synergistically complement each other. Our ears often fill in the cognitive blanks when our eyes are not entirely certain of what they are seeing and vice versa. You likely recall attending any number of social events or cocktail parties where everyone is conversing at once. Though we often can focus on a direct conversation, hearing a lot of dissonant, myriad sounds all at once can be distracting, even disorienting.

• **Behavioral**

You innately know that you should leave an area because of a loud, grating sound that is painful to listen to for an extended time, for instance, an obnoxious car alarm. What might not be as immediately apparent is that prolonged exposure can alter your disposition. Conversely, catchy music makes you want to get up and dance to the beat.

Even your choice of an alarm clock might negatively impact your mood for the day from the very time you get out of bed. There are far too many documented cases where a simple word or phrase has resulted in altercations costing friendships and relationships, altering the very fabric of life. It is not an exaggeration to note that words possess the power at their extreme to promote life or death.

Choosing the right sounds or music for an event will enhance the experience while significantly lengthening the time that attendees are engaged. Just as a filmmaker uses music, voices, and sound effects to set a mood or a tone for telling a story, one should be mindful when selecting the sounds and music used to complement the ambiance of an event. Proper soundscaping is paramount for retaining attendees during an event.

Education and Studying

Evidence suggests that background noise impacts students' ability to concentrate while studying. Whether it distracts them or enhances their focus largely depends on the individual's personality and the background noise's characteristics.

In terms of personality, introverts frequently grapple with concentrating when there is background noise. According to character studies, introverts struggle more on reading comprehension tests, memory tests, and mathematical tasks when background music or ambient office noise is present. They perform significantly better when there isn't any substantial background noise. The majority of introverts report feeling pressured and annoyed by background noise. They prefer to study or work on mental tasks in solitude, free from the interruptions that drain their psychological reserves.

However, regardless of the presence of background music or office noise, extroverts showed similar test results. Irrespective of whether background noise is present, it was noted that these individuals simply are unconcerned with ambient sound and function essentially the same either way.

The primary factor influencing how sound affects people while studying relates to how their brains are organized. The introvert's mental resources, which are optimized for memory recall and problem-solving, are essentially diverted by noise, which distracts them. For the extrovert, there is noticeably less blood flow to these brain regions. According to these results, extroverts don't tend to be as good at memory recall and problem-solving as introverts, but they function better in environments comprising numerous distractions. Extroverts also are believed to learn and retain information more effectively outside of a quiet environment. These mental types often find it challenging to focus in a quiet library setting because for them the silence is distracting.

Noise is typically thought to be disruptive to cognitive function. An additional element studied along these lines is syncopation, or the speed and beat of a noise that makes it audible, annoying, or distracting. For instance, the background noise in a library has a steady pace and beat that is largely regarded as pleasant to the ear. Electric fans that are running or the quiet noise an air conditioner makes deliver relatively constant noise levels, which typically is not too distracting. This consistency in sound level offers some measure of comfort to an introvert. There are also genres of music that are calming yet mentally stimulating and have been characterized as being able to improve academic performance.

On the flip side, unpredictable sounds and erratic tempos, such as intermittent traffic noises, can jolt the mental state. The brain then must make a concerted effort to return to its default state once the rhythm is disrupted.

Focusing can be difficult for those who find background noises distracting, possibly even intolerable, making learning and memorizing new information challenging. The solution for most of these individuals would be to reduce the noise level by wearing noise-canceling earplugs. This significantly lowers the volume of all ambient noise. If this is not sufficiently effective, alternatives would be incorporating a non-distracting soundtrack through the earpieces to override the ambient sounds or relocating to a less noisy environment if one is readily available.

Creativity

Given that certain music has been found to improve learning, memory, and cognition, it makes sense that the right music would also impact creative thinking. This premise is accurate in that music does help people think more creatively and flexibly, allowing them to shift between ideas and viewpoints rather than approaching a problem from a fixed vantage point.

Studies have shown that moderate audio inputs of roughly 70 dB during the generative phase of creative problem-solving help keep our idea gateway open and increase the chances of arriving at a final solution during the convergent phase.

Only some sounds, however, have been found by researchers to increase creative productivity. This does not include incessant noises, one-sided phone conversations, or abstract noises like white or pink noise. Contrarily, a cacophony of actual voices and other audible sounds from everyday life that fall within the acceptable range of 70 dB accomplishes this objective. Examples of beneficial sonic stimuli for creativity include the din of a busy cafe or the sound of rushing water.

Although the two halves of the brain have diverse functions from each other, they work together in concert. Our attempts to simplify something so infinitely complex as human cognition often lead to confusion about its respective functions. According to science, language processing occurs predominantly in the brain's left hemisphere. The right brain is used more frequently when performing tasks requiring movement, drawing, music, math, and technical skills.

The beauty of sound therapy is that it works on both hemispheres of the brain to strengthen areas that may be underdeveloped or to enhance communication function. At least ten different brain areas are activated just by listening to classical music. Language also draws on multiple brain regions in addition to the auditory cortex. As these connections are forged between many diverse segments of the brain, our creativity is embellished.

Marketing

A marketing tool, coined sound marketing, enables businesses to attract customers to their establishments by focusing on senses other than sight.

Sound is a powerful and essential component for making a business memorable to its customers. Sound marketing is included in this highly effective technique because every individual's behavior is directly influenced by every aspect of the senses, whether it be smell, hearing, touch, taste, or sight. Businesses have the opportunity to establish distinct promotional marketing strategies by appealing to these various sensory channels.

Thus, sound marketing becomes crucial, especially for businesses where customers cannot see the goods or services offered. Sound quality takes precedence over brand marketing in this scenario. Take, for instance, a customer calling a business; they cannot visualize the services offered. Still, effective sound marketing helps the company connect with the customer, essentially forging a sonic brand identity.

The competition from large companies with more powerful financial positions frequently overshadows startups and small businesses with limited resources. Therefore, these small businesses must find ways to compete in the same marketing space. Because of this, such companies now implement low-cost yet highly effective sound marketing strategies to increase customer satisfaction, brand awareness, and communication. Methods such as overhead announcements, background music, podcasts, and jingles have become widely implemented.

Entertainment

Sound is paramount for the entertainment industry because it engages viewers, aids information delivery, boosts production value, elicits emotional reactions, highlights what's on the screen, and conveys mood. The impact of creative output, including movies, music, and stage performances, is significantly influenced by the caliber and style of sound incorporated. When implemented effectively, language, sound effects, music, and even silence substantially improve video quality and impact. As importantly, poor audio will completely undermine an animation or video.

The best visual editing schemes will never be a substitute for or resolution to fixing poor sound implementation. Yet, conversely, sound cannot make up for poor animation, shoddy editing, or amateurish camera work. However, it is arguable that audio quality is more influential than video quality in terms of delivering a comprehensive audience experience. Sound enhances emotions and helps viewers relate to what they are seeing. It provides context for each image and cut scene while establishing the tone and mood of your story in its entirety.

For any production to have captivating audio, numerous factors must expertly be in place:

- Invest in top-notch equipment and a skilled sound operator.
- Record while monitoring the sound.
- Carefully select a location to minimize background noise.
- Mixing and mastering your sound is of utmost importance for the soundscape to work as a single cohesive unit.
- While editing, carefully ensure that the audio and video are perfectly synchronized.
- Establish a comprehensive, well-documented workflow to streamline editing.
- Work with an audio-savvy editor.

The quality of a video's picture is essential. Still, the sound is just as important, if not more so, to foster an unforgettable, immersive audience experience. When appropriately implemented, the three audio components of sound, music, and sound effects bring the finished work to life to effectively entertain, engage, and thrill the audience.

Soundscaping

Soundscaping is the preservation or enhancement of desired sounds while eliminating, suppressing, or masking undesirable sounds. This phrase is attributed to acousticians who research and construct sound environments appropriate to a specified objective. It describes the process of generating audio experiences relevant to a space's purpose, users, design, and intended brand experience.

Naturally, unwanted sounds vary from person to person and are entirely contextual. For example, it would be difficult to tolerate the kind of cluttered noise we would hear at a cocktail party while curled up with a good book at home. However, a similar level of commotion is expected in a coffee shop, where we manage to concentrate on and appreciate the same book.

Thus, soundscaping strives to maintain the appropriate sounds at the optimal levels in the designated place at the proper time. This is achieved by implementing the four components below.

1. Eliminating

This entails soundproofing, the process of building enclosures and barriers that prevent sound from transferring from the outside environment to a controlled internal space. This is achieved by meticulously enclosing areas.

On a slightly different plane, soundproofing can be attained on an individual basis controlling your personal sound environment. This can come in the form of devices like sound-canceling headphones or earbuds.

2. Suppressing

Suppression involves muting unwanted noises. Surfaces that absorb sound waves are used in those spaces to regulate which sound sources are truncated to minimize distraction when projecting desired sonic sources.

Sound suppressing is particularly important in spaces where high noise levels can be detrimental, such as recording studios, theaters, and residential buildings located near noisy environments. A more pleasant and controlled acoustic environment can be achieved by effectively controlling and suppressing unwanted noise, allowing for better focus, concentration, and sonic enjoyment.

3. Masking

To achieve this component, additional controlled sound is introduced into the environment. This methodology allows the brain to disregard background noises instead of being distracted by them, allowing the listener to concentrate on close-range conversations or tasks with an elevated level of privacy.

4. Diffusing

This is an entirely different approach that employs acoustic diffusers. Sound diffusion devices (diffusers and reflectors) are used to control sound in a given space by scattering and dispersing sound waves in different directions. This technique can be advantageous in large, complex rooms where traditional sound reinforcement techniques may be less effective. By carefully placing and adjusting sound diffusion devices, the overall acoustic characteristics of a space can be shaped, controlling factors such as reverberation time, frequency response, and spatial perception. This allows for creating customized acoustic environments that ultimately enhance the overall listening experience for audiences.

Designers use these four tools to control the noise inside and outside of a space. Whether or not the designer wants to improve the sound depends entirely on the experience they want to create and the tools they choose to use within the environment.

Sound Masking

Sound masking is a background noise specifically tuned to the same frequencies as human speech. It is utilized to attenuate certain sounds making them less discernible. While sound masking does not entirely eliminate these sounds, it does make conversations overheard from a distance more challenging to understand and less distracting.

Simply put, conversations that would typically be distracting to someone standing more than 15 feet away will be significantly less audible. Collaboration with coworkers in the immediate vicinity is not hindered by remote conversations because the distant conversations blend into the background. The added benefit is that speech privacy is enhanced.

Sound masking addresses noise distractions and speech privacy by lowering the speech intelligibility radius. Maintaining HIPAA compliance in hospitals and medical practices is a vital application of this technology. These facilities rely on sound masking to improve speech privacy and maintain patient confidentiality in exam rooms. Such sound regulating characteristics aid healthcare facility managers find it much simpler to create spaces where patient conversations won't be overheard. This technology also benefits intensive care units by helping patients rest while promoting healing.

Soundproofing

Soundproofing works in three ways;

1. Adding mass to a structure so that sound energy is reflected or transformed into heat, thereby blocking the noise.
2. Separating two structures so that sound vibrations cannot reach the second structure.
3. Sound absorption, which reduces the amount of sound that travels through a structure by absorbing sound (distributing the sound energy) through a material like Rockwool.

Soundproofing is like waterproofing; there can be no gaps. It's sound attenuating properties are only as strong as its weakest point. When soundproofing, it is essential to consider airborne noise and its impact.

Airborne sound is energy measured on a logarithmic scale in decibels. This scale measures the magnitude of sound energy; the energy level doubles for every increase of 3 dB measured. Since humans cannot easily detect increases of this magnitude, it is more efficient to use a scale stating that a 10 dB increase corresponds to a doubling of perceived noise. Therefore, this larger scale for dB reduction is more applicable for airborne noise.

Impact noise, also measured in decibels, determines how much impact energy a structure will transmit. Therefore, the lower the decibel value, the better the impact noise decibel rating.

The 30 to 40 dB range is a common target level for sound-proofing. This is considered a typical decibel rating for a standard domestic quiet room.

Ideally, readings are taken on both sides of the structure first, with noise being generated only on one side. This is to determine the level of soundproofing the existing structure inherently provides. A calculation then determines how much soundproofing material will be required to obtain the desired target rating to provide suitable peace and quiet.

The ideal soundproofing solution can be identified once the decibel levels are measured and compared with the desired target level. However, you might only have access to one side of the building in some circumstances. So, to calculate the target value, a sound decibel reading will be taken on the accessible side of the structure when the evaluation is determined to be at its loudest. This peak measure will be used as the background noise decibel level for the appropriate calculations.

Ambient Sound

Ambient sound is the term used to describe the background or surrounding noise for a specific setting. The sound of rain, birds singing, bees buzzing, and traffic hum all add to the ambiance.

It is often vital to hear ambient sounds while listening to your music. This enables you to remain aware of your surroundings. For instance, if you're out jogging on the streets, you should be mindful of the sound of approaching cars or other critical traffic sounds. Present-day technology allows for controlling ambient sounds.

In the work environment, background noise can have a negative impact on employee health because it can cause stress and possible hearing loss. According to studies, excessive noise levels are linked to increased workplace accidents because they impair workers' ability to exercise effective safety behaviors and recognize potential hazards by interfering with their ability to focus. This exposure and stress make employees more fatigued, leading to additional concerns. When appropriately used, noise-canceling headphones can effectively block out these sounds. These headphones are not always the ideal solution; whereas they can diminish stress and reduce the risk of hearing loss, they also decrease the sonic cues accompanying other safe work practices. A risk-versus-benefit evaluation and regard for federal, state, and local regulations are necessary to endorse a viable sound solution for work.

White Noise

White noise is sound containing equal energy at all frequencies within the sound spectrum of human hearing. It is often used as a sonic tool to provide various benefits, including:

Masking: White noise can mask or block out unwanted sounds by filling the auditory space with a consistent, neutral sound. This can help improve concentration and focus within noisy environments.

Relaxation: White noise's uniform and soothing quality can promote peace, helping reduce stress and anxiety.

Sleep: White noise can also aid sleep by creating a constant, predictable sound environment that can help mask irregular background noise, promoting a night of more restful sleep.

Tinnitus relief: People suffering from tinnitus often find relief while using white noise as it helps mask the ringing or buzzing sound they experience, reducing its impact.

Overall, there are several applications for white noise providing several sonic benefits, from masking unwanted noise to promoting relaxation and aiding sleep.

COUNTERING NOISE POLLUTION

Noise pollution is the term used to describe unwanted sound that has unpleasant effects and is annoying or painful to the ears. Noise pollution is typically produced by vehicles, horns, loudspeakers, planes, construction, etc. Usually, noise levels under 115 dB are bearable (within certain time parameters).

Noise pollution affects a significant number of people every day. Noise-induced hearing loss (NIHL) is the most frequent medical issue associated with it. Prolonged excessive noise exposure amplifies stress, heart disease, high blood pressure, and sleep disorders. All age groups, particularly children, are susceptible to these health issues. Numerous studies have shown that children living close to busy streets, railroads, or airports experience stress and other issues like memory, attention, and reading difficulties.

Although it is not as inherently harmful as air, water, or soil pollution, noise pollution is also regarded as an environmental threat. The effects of noise pollution over an extended period can be severe. It has an impact on the health and welfare of wildlife. Studies have shown that loud noises can make a caterpillar's dorsal vessel (an insects equivalent to a heart) beat more quickly and reduce the number of chicks that bluebirds produce. Animals use sound for numerous purposes, such as navigation, locating food, attracting mates, and fending off predators. These tasks are increasingly challenging for them because of noise pollution, impacting their capacity for survival.

By implementing the suggestions listed below, we can take action to reduce noise pollution.

- When not in use, turn off computers, TVs, video games, and other appliances around the house and office because they put unnecessary strain on the ears.
- To reduce repeated exposure to loud noises, shut the door after turning on dishwashers or washing machines

in the rooms where they are kept or turn them on before leaving the house.

- Put in earplugs to reduce loud noises to a tolerable level.
- Use headphones instead of speakers when listening to music, the radio, or TV, and keep the volume down to the minimal, functional level.
- Abide by noise level regulations for your area by environmental and health authorities.
- Respect quiet zones established near hospitals, schools, and other public places. Make sure noise limit signs are placed close to sensitive areas by taking appropriate action.
- Plant trees in your yard because they are effective for absorbing noise.
- Create soothing sounds in your home or workplace, i.e. music, singing birds, or waterfalls.
- Identify equipment that is producing noisy vibrations and take appropriate upkeep measures to reduce their volume and impact.
- Use proper lubrication and perform preventative maintenance to lessen friction between moving parts and keep the equipment operating at optimal performance.
- Inform the appropriate authorities if someone is violating noise level regulations.
- Frequently check interior and exterior noise levels for industrial complexes to ensure appropriate limits are maintained.

Doing our part in controlling the noises that are produced around us is essential. Spreading knowledge about noise pollution and its effects on people and the environment can begin with each of us.

Given what you now know, how do you want to take control of your sonic environment?

A PERSONAL JOURNEY

Be as simple as you can be; you will be astonished to see how uncomplicated and happy your life can become.

— PARAMAHANSA YOGANANDA

TRACK YOUR PROGRESS

It's time to put what you've learned into practice. Start experimenting in all facets of sound and music with regard to your physical, mental, and emotional well-being, as well as with your immediate surroundings and your active role in the field of sound. Keep a journal to record your experience.

Track your mood and physical state while listening to nature sounds, different music genres, MHz and binaural frequencies, etc. Note the personal effects and nuances of various sounds specific to you. Continue observing their influence for 12 hours following the sound experience. Record your responses expressly, both good and otherwise, positive and negative, towards diverse sound stimuli.

SOUND IN YOUR LIFE

As you've noted thus far, sound is an energy that has a wide range of applications. At this point, you might perceive sound as a whole new world of which you were previously largely unaware. Moreover, you may be somewhat uncertain of how to put everything you have learned into practice. The best course of action is always to break the process into manageable elements. Spend some time experimenting with sound in your life, whether once a day or once a week, as best suits your comfort level. Each time, concentrate on one aspect of your life. Ensure that you won't be distracted during this time.

Health and Well-Being

If your mental, physical, or emotional health lacks fulfillment, or if you feel under the weather in a general sense, consider experimenting with sound healing. With this experimentation, you're trying to determine what techniques and approaches best suit your needs so as to take advantage of these resources in the future or incorporate them into your regular routine. However, always seek qualified medical advice if you experience severe or persisting symptoms.

Physical Well-Being

You are now more fully aware of how various body organs respond to different sonic frequencies. Pay close attention to your physical state each day. Whenever you experience a headache or any other mild physical discomfort, review back to the principles covered in chapter five, "Sound Healing for the Body."

Revisit the frequencies for which each part of the body resonates. Online resources are readily available that offer the sounds corresponding to each resonating frequency. Binaural beats that fall within the necessary frequency range can be a part of this. Select a sound that feels fitting for the moment.

Each time you experiment, allow these sounds at least 30 minutes to take effect. Keep track of your physical, mental, and emotional state while being exposed to its influence immediately afterward and for several hours following. Some sounds will have little impact, while others will be significantly effective. Develop a chart, documenting solutions that effectively meet your needs for diverse circumstances and conditions. Then as you experience these physical discomforts you can easily and effectively tune into the frequencies that have proven beneficial.

Mental and Emotional Well-Being

Recognize your daily moods, whether consisting of stress, worry, anger, or sadness. Based on what you've learned, pay attention to the sounds recommended for specific emotional states. Furthermore, note any difficulties you may have falling asleep at night, especially if your mind is trapped in a state of racing thoughts. To review what you learned about how sound affects mental and emotional health, go back and reacquaint yourself with Chapter six, "Sound Healing for the Mind and Heart."

Find what works for you by experimenting with various approaches and sounds within the frequencies provided for each mental state. One such example is to revisit exposure to soothing music with native American, Celtic, and Indian stringed instruments, allowing you to relax when you are anxious. Alternatively, you could explore binaural beats more in-depth.

Recall your knowledge of brain wave frequencies and how to get the most from them. Submerse yourself in alpha brain wave frequencies, helping you relax when experiencing mild anxiety, and theta and delta brain wave frequencies to help you fall asleep when battling insomnia.

Once you've found a sound that speaks to you, give it 30–45 minutes of your time. Be mindful of any mood-altering effects this sound may elicit and savor its positive influence. Continue observing how you feel afterward to determine how long the results last. Write down your experience especially noting any particulars that will help you recreate these healing moments at will.

Mindfulness

Sound is a key factor in fostering mindfulness. Schedule 10 to 30 minutes for meditation every morning during the hour following waking. This is the time when you are still in touch with your subconscious self because your mind is in a theta state, again, the state which is halfway between sleep and wakefulness. This allows you to take fullest advantage of the ideal meditation period.

Include sound in your meditation routine. If you use guided meditations, look for sources that, in addition to the guiding voice, also feature healing sounds like nature sounds, binaural beats, bells, or singing bowls. Experiment with various methods, including mantras, chakra-balancing sounds, and affirmations. If you practice meditation independently, try doing so while immersed in healing sounds that encourage and enhance this period of introspection.

Create your own sound bath. You can accomplish this by locating a set of singing bowls or utilizing online resources that facilitate the sound bath experience.

Sound for Focus

Investigate how sound affects your ability to concentrate. As you have already learned, introverts and extroverts respond differently to ambient sonic stimuli. Test this theory to see if it holds true for you. Try listening to various sounds or musical genres while you work, noting their impact on your mental clarity and emotional status. Your experience may be completely different from the tenets included in this text; there are always exceptions to the rule.

With each healthful sound application you investigate, pay particular attention to your personal development recording your findings in writing.

Depending on the activity you are engaged in, a different type of sound may be more or less effective. Consider, for example, that while stimulating, upbeat music will most likely help you through boring or repetitive tasks, this same music will most certainly be a distraction when writing or conducting research. You may also discover that listening to classical music inspires creativity and increases productivity. Keep a detailed record of the traits of these sounds and how they affect each facet of the unique you.

- What is the activity?
- Which music or sounds best support this activity?
- What kind of music or sound interferes with this activity?
- Are they consistently effective, and if not, how long does the effect last?
- How long do they take to become effective?

Allow each sound to develop for at least 30 minutes. Depending on the day and how you are feeling, your responses might change. Each individual has distinct character and will therefore have diverse needs and reactions. Despite whatever the majority may appear to be, what genuinely matters is what works for you personally.

Sound at Your Workplace

Be mindful of the sounds around you when you are at your workplace. Is there a lot of noise and chatter that might be distracting? Perhaps there is a radio on. Are these noises preventing you from concentrating? Or does it instead improve your ability to focus? Is the ambient noise more subdued and obscure?

Certain offices have specific sound environments that encourage greater concentration than others. Given that the nature of your workplace permits it, if the sounds around you are distracting, get out your headphones and start experimenting. Analyze the sounds that help you be more productive at work. This could be soothing music, nature sounds, or recurrent and familiar songs from your playlist. In the event that you find silence to be the most effective setting, noise-canceling headphones may be your solution for increased productivity.

Look for opportunities that improve the ambient noise of your workplace. This can be an initiative you encourage for yourself along with your coworkers to create a more effective environment that benefits everyone.

Sound at Your Home

How would you describe the soundscape in your house? Do you find yourself often at peace, or do the surrounding sounds constantly make you want to seek escape?

If you have children, how do you involve music and sound in your interactions with them? Do you dance with them to inspiring music or sing them to sleep? What impact do these sounds have during those times?

What part does sound play in your relationship with your pets? What kinds of sounds elicit a reaction in your pets? Are there any noises that frighten or excite them?

Determine whether the predominant noises are positive or negative influences in your home. Hearing arguments or negative conversations around you affect how you feel in your body, your mood – your existence. Perhaps your next-door neighbor exhibits habits that are too loud. Evaluating and documenting any sounds you hear that either annoy or comfort you is important.

Deliberate how you can improve your home's sonic environment. Identify the sounds that help you relax and feel calm. Find ways to make these sounds more prevalent and adjust your routine to take advantage of them.

Sound for Special Occasions

When reaching important milestones or having memorable experiences, we often like to enhance these moments with just the right music. The sense of sound plays a significant role in these junctures and in preserving their memory.

Make notes or compose a journal of memories for special times when the sounds and music around you enhanced those moments. It could be a peaceful drive while listening to the ideal road music. It might be a freeing walk with the chirping of the birds and the sound of the leaves rustling all around. An occasion for celebration might be elevated by a particular musical highlight. Or, perhaps it's a New Year's Eve past, made even more memorable by the sound of friends gathered around, framed in vivid clarity because it was accompanied by the perfect music.

These sounds and music have the amazing ability to evoke strong emotions. Make a note of these feelings within you. What kind of music made you feel that way and why? How do you determine the ideal musical piece? What traits do you look for?

Endeavour to discover new, fascinating insights about yourself by keeping track of these sounds and music and exploring their role in your life. Keeping well-documented accounts will expedite the process, ensuring you save time when choosing the stellar background music for your next special occasion.

Expand on the knowledge presented within this book. Take advantage of the extensive "Reference" section at the end of this volume. These are not only provided to cite the resourced used to compile this work, but to provide you as the reader additional opportunity to further explore many facets of the sonic world that could only be introduced within the confines of these pages.

Devise how you're going to incorporate these experiments into your daily schedule. It all comes down to actively determining how you can apply the suggestions in this book to discover how sound and music can influence and enhance your overall well-being and quality of life.

CONCLUSION

When we are told that sound can influence us in many ways, we may not be too surprised because we experience it every day of our lives. However, what we have learned from our own experiences may only scratch the surface of the complex nature of sound and its potent influence. After reading this book, you have a solid understanding of this.

Sound has evolved throughout time, changing in form, character, and significance. Sound has been interpreted and used in many different ways over the years by everyone from shamanistic healers and spiritualists to scientists of the 20th century who realized sound is an energy that moves in waves. The use of sound in modern society spans a wide range of applications, including sonar technology for navigation, water filtration, music therapy, and healing.

Over and above words, the sounds we hear provide us with a wealth of information about the world and the things around us, including current events and whether or not we are safe. Sound healing is much more than just using singing bowls. Most of us would find life challenging in a world without sound. Everything is made of energy. All energy has a waveform. Those waveforms emit a frequency. An object's resonance is determined by this frequency.

The vibrations that makeup sound occur at the molecular level. These sound characteristics alter depending on whether the sound energy passes through a liquid, gas, or solid. These vibrations manifest in numerous fascinating ways. Sound can be represented as a visual entity through cymatics, which combines sound, geometry, light, and mathematics to produce stunning cymatic images in spheres, hexagons, and spirals. Although we may be unable to hear them, even plants use sound to communicate. These fascinating inaudible sounds of nature can now be accessed thanks to various methods and tools. These techniques have the potential to drastically alter people's lives by bridging new frontiers of the unknown, from spotting potential eruptions, storm trajectories, and nuclear tests to comprehending elephant behavior and bird communication.

The five different types of brain waves — gamma, beta, alpha, theta, and delta — are produced by electric currents that flow through the neurons in our brains. Each brain wave represents a different consciousness state, each supporting definitive activities while being unsuited for others. When we are aware of the multiple brain waves and their resonating frequencies, we can take steps to amplify them when we require them.

There are various ways to access these sounds, whether through tuning forks, meditation, sound baths, or any other instrument that makes healing sounds.

Trained professionals use music and sound in therapy to actively enhance and preserve a person's physical, psychological, and social well-being. Applying these methodologies is highly advantageous in assisting with managing mental and emotional complications such as anxiety, stress, sleep, and supporting physical well-being by enhancing memory, focus, blood circulation, immunity, and healthy cell activity. Most don't necessarily require the full resource of music therapy from a professional. In such cases, there are ways to incorporate its beneficial concepts into our daily lives for self-healing and enhancement of well-being, whether through music, nature sounds, binaural beats, or our own voice.

You already know in-depth how sound therapy can benefit physical health in a variety of ways, including treating skin conditions, insomnia, addiction, appetite and digestion, arthritis and rheumatism, aches and pains, sinuses, cancers, chronic fatigue, and many other disorders. We can take charge and select the strategies and resources to help us overcome any health-related challenge when we know and appropriately apply the resonating frequencies of each of our human organs.

Enhancing mental and emotional health can be accomplished successfully with music and sound therapy. It can aid in improving cognitive health, managing fear and anger, enhancing self-worth, and lowering depressive and negative thoughts. Each state of consciousness can be supported by the brain waves produced and regulated. Therefore, the more informed we are about which brain waves correspond to which mental and emotional states and what frequencies elicit those states, the more adept and proactive we can be in selecting the appropriate sound-healing methods.

Among the many benefits of sound is its ability to reach out to the soul and strengthen spiritual ties. There is a reason why sound and music are so important in religious rituals. It leads us toward harmony and establishes a direct channel with spirit. Music and sounds facilitate spiritual connection and convey ideas that, sometimes, cannot be expressed verbally. There are many ways that sound is incorporated into spiritual practices, specifically, but not limited to, hymns, chants, claps, sermons, and music. In shamanic rituals, the chakras are balanced using instruments such as singing bowls, gongs, drums, and tuning forks. Furthermore, sound serves as a guide for mantras, affirmations, and visualizations.

Sound is more complex than we may realize. This information should encourage us to pay closer attention to the sounds around us and how they influence us. The sound in an environment can either make or break the mood of any situation, whether it's a social gathering, while learning and studying, when being creative, for marketing, or for entertainment. Remember that sound does affect us physically, psychologically, cognitively, and behaviorally.

Although sound research still has room to advance, it has already made significant strides. There are impressive techniques for controlling the sounds around us today. You learned that sound scaping uses the methods of elimination, suppression, masking, and diffusion to manipulate the sonic environment in a given space. Uses for these technologies can be demonstrated by incorporating sound masking, which is helpful in offices and healthcare facilities, and soundproofing, which helps to lower noise pollution and is used extensively in the construction of recording studios.

Exploring the world of sound necessitates an understanding that noise pollution is a genuine concern. Human health can be negatively impacted by noise pollution. It can lead to stress, heart disease, high blood pressure, sleep disorders, and noise-induced hearing loss. Furthermore, it is detrimental to the health and welfare of wildlife as well as other aspects of nature. It is up to us to be the ones to educate ourselves, take the initiative to speak out, and do something about such issues.

Make use of the knowledge you have gained from this book in your daily life. Expand your understanding through your own research and explore the characteristics and benefits of sound more deeply. Experiment, keep track of your results, and make your own discoveries about the role that sound and music can become in your life. There is no limit to what we can discover about the world of sound. Therefore, take it slow and savor each experience. Allow this gift of sound and music to elevate your quality of life and well-being.

Despite the fact that we might or might not be aware of it, sound plays a significant role in our daily activities. When we explore this world, there are a lot of things to learn that can positively alter our lives. It can impact us in fascinating ways. Wherever we go, sound is all around us — even in the quietest of places.

Light and Sound are interwoven in the Language of Life.

— ELLE NICOLAI

BIBLIOGRAPHY

8 ways sound therapy can help you heal. (2022, March 18). Origins Lodge. https://originslodge.com/blog/8-ways-sound-therapy-can-help-you-heal/

Aakervik, A.-L. (2019, September 5). *Sound waves for your health.* Norwegian SciTech News. https://norwegianscitechnews.com/2019/09/sound-waves-for-your-health/

Abhang, P. A., Gawali, B. W., & Mehrotra, S. C. (2016). *Introduction to EEG- and speech-based emotion recognition.* Amsterdam Elsevier. https://www.elsevier.com/books/introduction-to-eeg-and-speech-based-emotion-recognition/abhang/978-0-12-804490-2 (Original work published 2022)

About us. (n.d.). Music of the Plants. Retrieved October 12, 2022, from https://www.musicoftheplants.com/about-us/

Acosta, C. (2021, May 2). *How to use sound baths for meditation and healing - sound bath singing bowl vibrations.* L'Officiel USA. https://www.lofficielusa.com/wellness/sound-baths-vibrational-meditation

Aggarwal, N. (2015). Brain healing sounds: Doctor designed: For study, meditation, memory, focus : 100% results! [YouTube Video]. In *YouTube.* https://www.youtube.com/watch?v=-8N9UR6OTCs

Altheia. (2015, January 26). Sound healing therapy: 14 mystical instruments that induce profound relaxation & inner quiet · lonerwolf. LonerWolf. https://lonerwolf.com/sound-healing-therapy/

Ambient sound. (2019). Media College. https://www.mediacollege.com/audio/ambient/

Amendolare, N. (2016). *What are sound waves? - definition, types & uses - video & lesson transcript | study.com.* Study.com. https://study.com/academy/lesson/what-are-sound-waves-definition-types-uses.html

American Heart Association. (2016, September 16). *Sound therapy may balance brain signals to reduce blood pressure, migraines.* MedicalXpress. https://medicalxpress.com/news/2016-09-therapy-brain-blood-pressure-migraines.html

American Music Therapy Association. (2005). *What is music therapy | what is music therapy? | american music therapy association (AMTA).* Music Therapy. https://www.musictherapy.org/about/musictherapy/

An introduction to crystal sound healing | what is crystal sound healing? (2011, December 16). Natural Therapy Pages. https://www.naturaltherapypages. com.au/article/an_introduction_to_crystal_sound_healing

Anxiety and sound therapy. (2017, August 17). US Version | Sound Therapy. https://mysoundtherapy.com/us/what-is-sound-therapy/emotional-stress-relief/anxiety/

Arnaud, J. (2022, July 1). *What are binaural beats and how can they help you focus?* The Los Angeles Film School. https://www.lafilm.edu/blog/what-are-binaural-beats-and-how-can-they-help-you-focus/

Arnold, L. (2014, November 23). *How sound affects you: Cymatics, an emerging science.* Ask.Audio; Ask.Audio. https://ask.audio/articles/how-sound-affects-you-cymatics-an-emerging-science

Auto, F. M. L., Amancio, O. M. S., & Lanza, F. de C. (2015). The effect of music on weight gain of preterm infants older than 32 weeks: a randomized clinical trial. *Revista Paulista de Pediatria, 33,* e293–e299. https://doi.org/10. 1590/0103-058231369512

Awika, R. (2020, October 8). *How to heal your mind and body with powerful sounds.* Medium. https://medium.com/illumination/how-to-heal-your-mind-and-body-with-powerful-sounds-c8ee64a1dbd

Benton, M. (2016). *Gong therapy: Sound, healing & yoga.* Bookshelf Press.

Bettine, M. (2016, May 17). *Sound is the medicine of forever.* Sound Is the Medicine of Forever. http://thewayofthegong.blogspot.com/2016/05/sound-is-medicine-of-forever.html

Bhaumik, G. (2019, December 27). *Sound healing explained - how it works and health benefits.* Destination Deluxe. https://destinationdeluxe.com/sound-healing-health-benefits/

Binaural beats for anxiety | bettersleep. (2022, April 13). BetterSleep. https:// www.bettersleep.com/blog/binaural-beats-for-anxiety/

Birds may use "sound maps" to navigate huge distances. (2013, February 1). NPR. https://www.npr.org/2013/02/01/170884694/birds-may-use-sound-maps-to-navigate-huge-distances

Boost self confidence with 528hz - the frequency of transformation. (2017, April 10). Meditative Mind. https://meditativemind.org/boost-self-confidence-with-528hz-the-frequency-of-transformation/

Boothby, S. (2017, April 13). *How does music affect your mood and emotions.* *Healthline.* https://www.healthline.com/health-news/mental-listening-to-music-lifts-or-reinforces-mood-051713

Borchard, T. J. (2018, January 28). *Words can change your brain.* Psych Central. https://psychcentral.com/blog/words-can-change-your-brain-2#2

Boyd-Brewer, C., & McCaffrey, R. (2004). *Vibroacoustic sound therapy improves pain management and more.* Holistic Nursing Practice, 18(3), 111–118. https://doi.org/10.1097/00004650-200405000-00002

Brainwave frequencies and effects. (n.d.). NeuroSonica. Retrieved October 26, 2022, from https://www.neurosonica.com/the-science/brainwave-types-frequencies.html

Brazier, Y. (2016, March 20). *Crunch effect: How the sounds of eating curb the appetite.* Medical News Today. https://www.medicalnewstoday.com/articles/308060#People-eat-more-if-they-cannot-hear-their-own-chewing

Brenizer, M. (2018, March 29). *The power of sound meditation - all you need to know.* DoYou. https://www.doyou.com/what-is-sound-meditation-and-why-is-it-so-trendy-38218/

Brennan, D. (2021, April 12). *What are binaural beats?* WebMD. https://www.webmd.com/balance/what-are-binaural-beats

Brill, P. (2021, May 27). *Evaluating the advantages of sound therapy sessions in mental and physical health | pearlbrill.* Pearlbrill. https://pearlbrill.com/evaluating-advantages-sound-therapy-sessions-mental-and-physical-health

Brut India. (2021, September 30). *Artist invents device that can listen to plant music.* YouTube. https://www.youtube.com/watch?v=VMvSAjkQg9I

Buzz Staff. (2021, September 30). *It's 2021 and you can now listen to music made by plants.* News18. https://www.news18.com/news/buzz/its-2021-and-you-can-now-listen-to-music-made-by-plants-4265087.html

Cafasso, J. (2017, October 6). *Do binaural beats have health benefits?* Healthline; Healthline Media. https://www.healthline.com/health/binaural-beats

Can background noise actually help you study better? (2018, August 13). Online Schools Center. https://www.onlineschoolscenter.com/can-background-noise-actually-help-you-study-better/

Can music help you deal with negativity? | incadence music therapy blog. (n.d.). Incadence. Retrieved October 25, 2022, from https://www.incadence.org/post/can-music-help-you-deal-with-negativity

Cast out negative thoughts by coloring on music beats. (2020, May 28). Branding News. https://www.branding.news/2020/05/28/cast-out-negative-thoughts-by-coloring-on-music-beats/

Chase. (2015, July 18). *Studies confirm "sound therapy" can aid arthritis, cancer, tinnitus, autoimmune disease and more using vibrational frequencies & deep relaxation. ISTA.* https://istasounds.org/studies-confirm-sound-therapy-heals-arthritis-cancer-tinnitus-autoimmune-disease-and-more-using-vibrational-frequencies/

Chronic Pain and Sound Therapy. (n.d.). US Version | Sound Therapy. Retrieved October 23, 2022, from https://mysoundtherapy.com/us/what-is-sound-therapy/emotional-stress-relief/chronic-pain/#:~:text=Sound%20Therapy%20uses%20highly%20filtered

Cleveland Clinic. (2020, November 24). *Music therapy: What is it, types & treatment.* Cleveland Clinic. https://my.clevelandclinic.org/health/treatments/8817-music-therapy

Clohessy, L. (2018). Music therapy and mental health | lucia clohessy | tedxwcmephamhigh [YouTube Video]. In *YouTube.* https://www.youtube.com/watch?v=-io-uld2JFU

Cooper, L. (2016, October 6). *Top four ways to improve your creativity with sound.* The British Academy of Sound Therapy. https://www.britishacademyofsoundtherapy.com/top-4-ways-improve-creativity/

Cooper, L. (2017, September 3). *A natural way to ease migraine.* The British Academy of Sound Therapy. https://www.britishacademyofsoundtherapy.com/migraine/

Creativity and sound therapy. (2018, December 18). US Version | Sound Therapy. https://mysoundtherapy.com/us/what-is-sound-therapy/brain-performance/creativity/

Cross, A. (2020, December 22). *Who knew that plants make music? Here's a device that allows you to hear them.* Alan Cross' a Journal of Musical Things. https://www.ajournalofmusicalthings.com/who-knew-that-plants-make-music-heres-a-device-that-allows-you-to-hear-them/

Depression and sound therapy. (n.d.). US Version | Sound Therapy. Retrieved October 25, 2022, from https://mysoundtherapy.com/us/what-is-sound-therapy/emotional-stress-relief/depression/#:~:text=Sound%20Therapy%20has%20been%20found

Dorfner, M. (2018, April 24). *Don't ignore these 7 serious symptoms.* Mayo Clinic News Network. https://newsnetwork.mayoclinic.org/discussion/dont-ignore-these-7-serious-symptoms/

Duarte, M. L. M., & de Brito Pereira, M. (2006). Vision influence on whole-body human vibration comfort levels. *Shock and Vibration,* 13(4-5), 367–377. https://doi.org/10.1155/2006/950682

Durkin, P. (2017, March 23). *Dr. masaru emoto and water consciousness.* Structured Water Superstore. https://thewellnessenterprise.com/emoto/

Early, J. (1997, June 25). *Sacred sounds: Belief & society.* Smithsonian Music. https://music.si.edu/story/sacred-sounds-belief-society

Energy and sound therapy. (2018, December 13). US Version | Sound Therapy. https://mysoundtherapy.com/us/what-is-sound-therapy/emotional-stress-relief/energy-fatigue/

Enlightened solutions - why is sound therapy effective for addiction treatment? (2017, May 26). Enlightened Solutions. https://enlightenedsolutions.com/why-is-sound-therapy-effective-for-addiction-treatment/

EntheoNation. (n.d.). *What is shamanic sound healing? – entheonation.* Entheonation. Retrieved October 3, 2022, from https://entheonation.com/blog/shamanic-sound-healing/

Eveleth, R. (2016, January 5). *What did the big bang sound like?* The Atlantic. https://www.theatlantic.com/science/archive/2016/01/a-brief-history-of-noise/422481/

Fetyan, N. A. H., & Salem Attia, T. M. (2020). Water purification using ultra-sound waves: Application and challenges. *Arab Journal of Basic and Applied Sciences,* 27(1), 194–207. https://doi.org/10.1080/25765299.2020.1762294

Gabriel, R. (2015, January 15). *How to use sound to heal yourself.* Chopra. https://chopra.com/articles/how-to-use-sound-to-heal-yourself

Gagliano, M. (2012). Green symphonies: A call for studies on acoustic communication in plants. *Behavioral Ecology,* 24(4), 789–796. https://doi.org/10.1093/beheco/ars206

Gagliano, M., Mancuso, S., & Robert, D. (2012). Towards understanding plant bioacoustics. *Trends in Plant Science,* 17(6), 323–325. https://doi.org/10.1016/j.tplants.2012.03.002

Gallagher, A. (2020, January 9). *Does sound therapy actually help relieve migraines?* National Headache Institute. https://nationalheadacheinstitute.com/blog/does-sound-therapy-actually-help-relieve-migraines/#:~:text=White%20noise%20is%20essentially%20background

Gherini, A. (2017, November 20). *How the beach benefits your brain, according to science.* Inc.; Inc. https://www.inc.com/anne-gherini/how-beach-benefits-your-brain-according-to-science.html

Gibson, D. (2011, October 13). *How sound affects us physically, mentally, emotionally and spiritually.* Sound Travels. https://www.soundtravels.co.uk/a-How_Sound_Affects_us_Physically,_Mentally,_Emotionally_and_Spiritually-541.aspx

Gillihan, S. J. (2019, November 16). *How to improve anxiety, sleep, and more with binaural beats | psychology today south africa.* Psychology Today. https://www.psychologytoday.com/za/blog/think-act-be/201911/how-improve-anxiety-sleep-and-more-binaural-beats

Gould, W. R. (2020, June 30). *What are sound baths?* Verywell Mind. https://www.verywellmind.com/what-are-sound-baths-4783501

Goveya, W. (2018, May 22). *Music therapy: A medium for communication and love.* TED. https://www.ted.com/talks/wyomia_goveya_music_therapy_a_medium_for_communication_and_love?utm_campaign=tedspread&utm_medium=referral&utm_source=tedcomshare

Grant, K. (2021, September 30). *How sound therapy & sound baths can help people learn to stop stress eating.* In Fitness and in Health. https://medium.com/in-fitness-and-in-health/how-sound-therapy-sound-baths-can-help-people-learn-to-stop-stress-eating-5276341d91b8

Green Queen Team. (2022, May 1). *Bioacoustics: Listening to nature is our only option to solve the climate crisis.* Green Queen. https://www.greenqueen.com.hk/bioacoustics-listening-to-nature/

Greenwood, M. (2022, May 25). *People swear this type of music helps anxiety—but does it really work?* Self. https://www.self.com/story/binaural-beats-benefits

Grossman, C. (2020, August 3). *Sound and spirit: Music as a path to awakening.* Insight Timer Blog. https://insighttimer.com/blog/sound-and-spirit-music-as-a-path-to-awakening/

Hagstrum, J. T. (2001). Infrasound and the avian navigational map. *Journal of Navigation, 54*(3), 377–391. https://doi.org/10.1017/s037346330100145x

Hales, D. (2021, February 2). *Cheapest way to soundproof a room.* Modern Castle. https://moderncastle.com/blog/cheapest-way-to-soundproof-a-room/

Harrison, P. (2019, August 8). *13 best sound healing instruments for therapy.* The Daily Meditation Coaching Sessions. https://www.thedailymeditation.com/sound-healing-everything-you-need-to-know-about-healing-sounds

Harvard Health Publishing. (2015, February 14). *Music can boost memory and mood - harvard health.* Harvard Health; Harvard Health. https://www. health.harvard.edu/mind-and-mood/music-can-boost-memory-and-mood

Hassanien, R. H., Hou, T., Li, Y., & Li, B. (2014). Advances in effects of sound waves on plants. *Journal of Integrative Agriculture,* 13(2), 335–348. https:// doi.org/10.1016/s2095-3119(13)60492-x

Healing frequencies of the human body: Full list and benefits. (2020, March 21). Mind Is the Master. https://mindisthemaster.com/sound-frequency-healing-human-body-benefits/

Healing Waves. (n.d.). Deep sleep - eczema relief. Insight Timer. Retrieved October 22, 2022, from https://insighttimer.com/healingwaves/guided-meditations/deep-sleep-eczema-relief

Henning, D., Sabic, E., & Hout, M. C. (2018). Hear and there: Sounds from everywhere! *Frontiers for Young Minds,* 6. https://doi.org/10.3389/frym. 2018.00063

High intensity focused ultrasound | other treatments | cancer research UK. (2022, June 22). Cancer Research UK. https://www.cancerresearchuk.org/about-cancer/cancer-in-general/treatment/other/high-intensity-focused-ultrasound-hifu#:~:text=HIFU%20is%20a%20cancer%20treatment

History. (2021, March 24). Music of the Plants. https://www.musicoftheplants. com/history/

Ho, S. (2022, September 3). *Sound therapy: What it is, how to practice it, and where to find it.* Green Queen. https://www.greenqueen.com.hk/what-is-sound-healing-therapy/#:~:text=These%20include%20listening%20to% 20music

Holmes, I. (2002). Sound cleans up water purification. *Nature.* https://doi.org/ 10.1038/news020413-4

Holmes, O. W. (1888). *Over the teacups.* Houghton, Mifflin and Co. https:// www.gutenberg.org/files/2689/2689-h/2689-h.htm

How do sound and matter interact? | study.com. (2020). Study.com. https://study. com/academy/lesson/how-do-sound-and-matter-interact.html

How to reduce noise pollution? (2017, June 8). Perfect Pollucon Services. https:// www.ppsthane.com/blog/how-to-reduce-noise-pollution

Howland, K. M. (2015). How music can heal our brain and heart | Kathleen M. Howland | TedxBerkleeValencia [YouTube Video]. In *YouTube.* https:// www.youtube.com/watch?v=NIY4yCsGKXU

Infrasound monitoring | CTBTO. (n.d.). CTBTO. Retrieved October 16, 2022, from https://www.ctbto.org/our-work/monitoring-technologies/infra sound-monitoring#:~:text=The%20IMS%20infrasound%20network%20is

Insight timer - #1 free meditation app for sleep, relax & more. (n.d.). Insighttimer.-com. Retrieved October 18, 2022, from https://insighttimer.com/medita tion-topics/soundmeditation

Jernigan, C. (2021, January 17). *How music therapy can help with anger manage-ment | incadence music therapy blog.* Incadence. https://www.incadence.org/post/how-music-therapy-can-help-with-anger-management

Julious, B. (2020, June 10). *The sound solution. Cancer Wellness.* https://cancer wellness.com/complementary-medicine/sound-gong-therapy-medita tion-cancer/

Kelley, A. (2018, August 27). *The importance of sound and how it can transform an event experience.* GES. https://insights.ges.com/us-blog/importance-of-sound-and-how-it-can-transform-an-event-experience

Khait, I., Lewin-Epstein, O., Sharon, R., Saban, K., Perelman, R., Boonman, A., Yovel, Y., & Hadany, L. (2018). *Plants emit informative airborne sounds under stress.* https://doi.org/10.1101/507590

Khan, H. I. (1996). *The mysticism of sound and music.* Shambhala ; [New York. http://www.hazrat-inayat-khan.org/php/views.php?h1=10&h2=17

Kim, H.-W., Roh, D.-H., Yoon, S.-Y., Kang, S.-Y., Kwon, Y.-B., Han, H.-J., Lee, H.-J., Choi, S.-M., Ryu, Y.-H., Beitz, A. J., & Lee, J.-H. (2006). The anti-inflammatory effects of low- and high-frequency electroacupuncture are mediated by peripheral opioids in a mouse air pouch inflammation model. *Journal of Alternative and Complementary Medicine* (New York, N.Y.), 12(1), 39–44. https://doi.org/10.1089/acm.2006.12.39

Kiniry, L. (2013, July 18). *5 things we can learn from sounds we can't hear.* Popular Mechanics. https://www.popularmechanics.com/science/environment/g1246/5-things-we-can-learn-from-sounds-we-cant-hear/?slide=5

Kiniry, L. (2014, March 17). *7 amazing things you can do with sound waves.* Popular Mechanics; Popular Mechanics. https://www.popularmechanics. com/military/g1458/7-amazing-things-you-can-do-with-sound-waves/?slide=1

Knowlton, C. (2017, August 1). *Sonar technology.* Discovery of Sound in the Sea. https://dosits.org/galleries/technology-gallery/locating-objects-using-sonar/sonar/

Krause, A. M. (2019, November 7). *When plants sing: Plant bioacoustics and the problem of anthropomorphism - adam michael krause*. Harbinger. https://harbinger-journal.com/issue-1/when-plants-sing/

Lambert, J. M., Bloom, S. E., Nickerson, C. M., Clay, C. J., & Samaha, A. L. (2019). Evaluating functional differences between positive and negative reinforcement through preference for parameters of sound manipulation. *Revista Mexicana de Análisis de La Conducta*, 45(2), 173–198. https://www.redalyc.org/journal/593/59367995002/html/

LaTour, M. (2020, March 5). *Interesting ways that sound waves are used*. Soundwave Art. https://soundwaveart.com/interesting-ways-that-sound-waves-are-used/

Lerner, L. (2021, August 28). *Sound energy: Everything you need to know*. Just Energy. https://justenergy.com/blog/sound-energy-everything-you-need-to-know/

Lhamo, L. (2019, May 27). *Sound harmony sacred geometry*. Yoga Alliance Professionals. https://blog.yogaallianceprofessionals.org/sound-harmony-sacred-geometry

Li, K., Weng, L., & Wang, X. (2021). *The state of music therapy studies in the past 20 years: A bibliometric analysis*. Frontiers in Psychology, 12. https://doi.org/10.3389/fpsyg.2021.697726

Lifestyle Staff. (2022, February 22). *Struggling with stress and anxiety/ try sound therapy to calm and heal the mind* (A. Thakur, Ed.). India. https://www.india.com/health/struggling-with-stress-and-anxiety-try-sound-therapy-to-calm-and-heal-the-mind-5251713/

Long, R. (2020, November 3). *The benefits of sound meditation*. Mirosuna. https://mirosuna.com/blog/the-benefits-of-sound-meditation/#:~:text=Sound%20meditation%20is%20the%20use

Louart, C. (2016, July 10). *Music to heal memory*. CNRS News. https://news.cnrs.fr/articles/music-to-heal-memory

Lyxell, B., Wass, M., Sahlén, B., Ibertsson, T., Asker-Árnason, L., Uhlén, I., Henricson, C., Mentzer, C. V., Mäki-Torkko, E., & Möller, C. (2013). *Hearing and cognitive development in deaf and hearing-impaired children*. ScienceDirect; Elsevier. https://www.sciencedirect.com/topics/biochemistry-genetics-and-molecular-biology/auditory-stimulation

Macmillan, A. (2017, March 8). *The sound of "pink noise" improves sleep and memory*. Time. https://time.com/4694555/pink-noise-deep-sleep-improve-memory/

Martinez, N. (2015, February 19). *What you need to know about sound healing.* MindBodyGreen. https://www.mindbodygreen.com/articles/sound-healing

Massad, S. (n.d.). *What is untherapy?* Retrieved October 2, 2022, from http://www.menumill.com/assets/0001/8529/What_is_UnTherapy_.pdf

Mayberry, M. (2015, October 2). *Your words have impact, so think before you speak.* Entrepreneur. https://www.entrepreneur.com/leadership/your-words-have-impact-so-think-before-you-speak/251290

McCumiskey, C. (2020, June 13). *Words can affect your brain functions.* Independent. https://www.independent.ie/regionals/corkman/lifestyle/words-can-affect-your-brain-functions-39280807.html

McMorrow, B. (n.d.). *Five ways chanting heals us.* Kripalu. Retrieved October 20, 2022, from https://kripalu.org/resources/five-ways-chanting-heals-us

Meda, K. (2019, November 26). *How to manipulate brain waves for a better mental state.* The Nexus. https://nexus.jefferson.edu/science-and-technology/how-to-manipulate-brain-waves-for-a-better-mental-state/

Meissner, M. (2022, April 12). *Music therapy and eczema: What to know.* Medical News Today. https://www.medicalnewstoday.com/articles/can-music-therapy-treat-eczema#summary

Merz, B. (2015, November 4). *Healing through music.* Harvard Health Blog. https://www.health.harvard.edu/blog/healing-through-music-201511058556

Mirzaei, N. (2020, December 16). *The spiritual nature of shamanic drumming.* Meditation Music Library. https://meditationmusiclibrary.com/blogs/wednesday-wisdom-blog/the-spiritual-nature-of-shamanic-drumming

Muse. (2018, June 25). *A deep dive into brainwaves: Brainwave frequencies explained.* Muse. https://choosemuse.com/blog/a-deep-dive-into-brain waves-brainwave-frequencies-explained-2/

Music can heal your skin. (2021, January 13). Navinka. https://www.navinkaskin.com/blogs/skin-talk-1/music-can-heal-your-skin

Music therapy. (2015). Good Therapy. https://www.goodtherapy.org/learn-about-therapy/types/music-therapy

Music therapy: What is it, types & treatment. (2020, November 24). Cleveland Clinic. https://my.clevelandclinic.org/health/treatments/8817-music-therapy

Nathanson, J. A., & Berg, R. E. (2018). Noise pollution | definition, examples, control, & facts. In *Encyclopædia Britannica.* https://www.britannica.com/science/noise-pollution

National Oceanic and Atmospheric Administration. (n.d.). *What is sonar?* Oceanservice.noaa.gov. Retrieved October 4, 2022, from https://oceanservice.noaa.gov/facts/sonar.html#:~:text=Sonar%20uses%20sound%20waves%20to%20

New international monitoring system map launched | CTBTO. (n.d.). CTBTO. Retrieved October 16, 2022, from https://www.ctbto.org/news-and-events/news/new-international-monitoring-system-map-launched

Nicolai, E. (n.d.). *Light language quotes (2 quotes).* Goodreads. Retrieved November 5, 2022, from https://www.goodreads.com/quotes/tag/light-language

Noise pollution - definition, types, causes, prevention. (n.d.). BYJUS. Retrieved November 2, 2022, from https://byjus.com/physics/noise-pollution-prevention/#Prevention

Noise pollution | national geographic society. (2022). National Geographic. https://education.nationalgeographic.org/resource/noise-pollution

Novotney, A. (2013, November). *Music as medicine.* American Psychological Association, 46. https://www.apa.org/monitor/2013/11/music

Opinion, & Horton, L. (2019, August 8). *The neuroscience behind our words.* BRM Institute. https://brm.institute/neuroscience-behind-words/

Oralde, T. (2022, February 1). *What is ambient sound? [Everything you wanted to know].* Electric Field Festival. https://electricfieldsfestival.com/what-is-ambient-sound/

Page, D. (2022, March 7). *The effects of music on metabolism, even when you're sitting - audio factor.* Audio Factor. https://audio-factor.com/weight-loss-music/49-effects-of-music/

Pardes, A. (2019, September 25). *Let your plants play music, and gardens of sound will bloom.* Wired. https://www.wired.com/story/plantwave-music/

Patnaik, T. (2021, August 20). *Sound healing | sound therapy.* MedIndia. https://www.medindia.net/patients/lifestyleandwellness/sound-healing.htm#what-is-sound-healing

Patrick, S. C., Assink, J. D., Basille, M., Clusella-Trullas, S., Clay, T. A., den Ouden, O. F. C., Joo, R., Zeyl, J. N., Benhamou, S., Christensen-Dalsgaard, J., Evers, L. G., Fayet, A. L., Köppl, C., Malkemper, E. P., Martín López, L. M., Padget, O., Phillips, R. A., Prior, M. K., Smets, P. S. M., & van Loon, E. E. (2021). Infrasound as a cue for seabird navigation. *In Frontiers in Ecology and Evolution* (Vol. 9). https://doi.org/10.3389/fevo.2021.740027

Paul, M. (2017, August 15). *Sound waves enhance deep sleep and memory. Northwestern Now.* https://news.northwestern.edu/stories/2017/april/pink-noise-sound-enhance-deep-sleep-memory/

Peralta, L. (2021, November 3). *Impact of music on society - sociological effects.* Save the Music Foundation. https://www.savethemusic.org/blog/how-does-music-affect-society/#:~:text=How%20does%20music%20affect%20our

Plant bioacoustics. (2022, April 17). Wikipedia. https://en.wikipedia.org/wiki/Plant_bioacoustics#:%7E:text=Plants%20emit%20audio%20acoustic%20emissions

Priyadarshi, S. (2019, August 2). *Introduction: Understanding the functions of sounds in our everyday lives.* Sound Experience Design. https://medium.com/sound-experience-design/introduction-understanding-the-func tions-of-sounds-in-our-everyday-lives-b7eb168e14cf

Pujol, R. (2018, June 6). *Journey into the world of hearing - specialists.* Cochlea. http://www.cochlea.org/en/hear/human-auditory-range#:%7E:text= Human%20ear%20perceives%20frequencies%20between

Purves, D., Augustine, G. J., Fitzpatrick, D., Katz, L. C., Anthony-Samuel LaMantia, McNamara, J. O., & S Mark Williams. (2018). *The audible spectrum.* NCBI; Sinauer Associates. https://www.ncbi.nlm.nih.gov/books/NBK10924/

Rattner, D. M. (2017, June 23). *How noise can improve your creativity.* Medium. https://medium.com/s/how-to-design-creative-workspaces/how-noise-can-improve-your-creativity-980bd82f278#:~:text=Under%20the%20right%20circumstances%2C%20a

Releasing stress through the power of music | counseling services | university of nevada, reno. (2022). University of Nevada, Reno. https://www.unr.edu/counseling/virtual-relaxation-room/releasing-stress-through-the-power-of-music

Rettner, R. (2016, September 16). *How "brainwave-balancing" therapy could ease migraines.* Live Science. https://www.livescience.com/56121-brainwave-balancing-hirrem-migraines.html

Rossman, M. L., Wexler, J., & Oyle, I. (1974). The use of sonopuncture in some common clinical syndromes. *The American Journal of Chinese Medicine,* 02(02), 199–201. https://doi.org/10.1142/s0192415x74000250

Ryan, D. (2018, March 19). *Sound healing facials.* The Facial Goddess. https://www.thefacialgoddess.com/sound-healing-facials/

Ryan, T. (2021, June 22). *Binaural beats for sleep.* Sleep Foundation. https://www.sleepfoundation.org/noise-and-sleep/binaural-beats

S, T. (2022, January 5). *The ultimate guide to tuning fork healing with sound therapy in 2022.* Lots of Zen. https://lotsofzen.com/blogs/news/tuning-fork-healing-with-sound-therapy#:~:text=There%20are%20two%20types%20of

Sacks, O. (2012). *Awakenings.* Picador. (Original work published 1973)

Sadeghi, H. (2014, May 29). *The power of words: How words affect our lives | Goop.* Goop. https://goop.com/wellness/mindfulness/the-scary-power-of-negative-words/

Santos-Longhurst, A. (2018a). *Sound healing 101: What is it and how does it work?* Healthline. https://www.healthline.com/health/sound-healing

Santos-Longhurst, A. (2018b, July 18). *Music as therapy: The uses and benefits of sound healing.* Healthline; Healthline Media. https://www.healthline.com/health/sound-healing#types

Satchidananda, S. (2012, July 21). *"The relationship between prana & sound" - A talk by swami satchidananda.* YouTube; Integral Yoga. https://www.youtube.com/watch?v=U1fhWMCMDr8&t=416s

Schultz, C. (2014, January 8). *Expose wounds to the right kind of sounds, and they heal faster.* Smithsonian Magazine. https://www.smithsonianmag.com/smart-news/expose-wounds-to-the-right-kind-of-sounds-and-they-heal-faster-180949295/

Science of soundproofing - ikoustic soundproofing. (2022, June 29). IKoustic. https://www.ikoustic.co.uk/science-soundproofing/

Sound. (n.d.). Science World. Retrieved October 5, 2022, from https://www.scienceworld.ca/resource/sound/#:~:text=Sound%20is%20a%20type%20of

Scott, T. (2021, August 20). *Frequencies + the body.* Health & Bass. https://www.healthandbass.com/post/frequencies-and-the-body

Sengar, C. (2022, July 19). *How sound therapy can help aid physical and mental health conditions.* Onlymyhealth. https://www.onlymyhealth.com/sound-therapy-for-physical-mental-problems-1658211896

Serani, D. (2020, May 23). *Binaural beats music can reduce depression.* Psychology Today. https://www.psychologytoday.com/us/blog/two-takes-depression/202005/binaural-beats-music-can-reduce-depression

Shabnam, J., Mahsa, A., Manoochehr, M., & Sonia, O. (2021). Effect of music on the growth monitoring of low birth weight newborns. *International Journal of Africa Nursing Sciences,* 14, 100–312. https://doi.org/10.1016/j.ijans.2021.100312

Shamanic sound healing / shamanic sound healing. (2019, June 25). Shamanic Sound Healing. https://shamanicsoundhealing.com/shamanic-sound-healing/

Sharma, A. (2022, August 31). *How to use sound to heal yourself - times of india.* The Times of India. https://timesofindia.indiatimes.com/life-style/health-fitness/home-remedies/how-to-use-sound-to-heal-yourself/articleshow/93899053.cms

Sharma, M. (2018, December 20). *How sound therapy can help manage stress and depression? - by dr. manan sharma.* Lybrate. https://www.lybrate.com/topic/how-sound-therapy-can-help-manage-stress-and-depression/38241247e480853e87473cde7e672c5f

Sharpe, L. (2015, July 16). *Sound waves could speed up wound healing.* Popular Science. https://www.popsci.com/sound-waves-accelerate-healing/

Sharratt, A. (2019, October 16). *Good vibrations: The healing power of sound.* The Globe and Mail. https://www.theglobeandmail.com/life/article-good-vibrations-the-healing-power-of-sound/?page=all

Sheridan, K. (Director). (2007). *August Rush* [Film]. Warner Bros. Pictures & Odyssey Entertainment.

Shoemaker, C. (2016). *The power of sound: Soundwaves, brainwaves, and binaural beats / sanesco health.* Sanesco. https://sanescohealth.com/blog/the-power-of-sound-soundwaves-brainwaves-and-binaural-beats/

Singing bowls for beginners: The complete guide (updated 2022). (2019, November 18). Shanti Bowl. https://www.shantibowl.com/blogs/blog/singing-bowls-for-beginners-the-complete-guide

Skin healing sound frequencies. healing sounds for skin disease. (n.d.). Sound Your Illness Away. Retrieved October 22, 2022, from https://sound-pharmacy.com/product-category/skin/

Sleep, insomnia and sound therapy. (2017, August 17). US Version | Sound Therapy. https://mysoundtherapy.com/us/what-is-sound-therapy/emotional-stress-relief/sleep-insomnia/

Smith, D. G. (2020, March 3). *How to hack your brain with sound.* Medium. https://elemental.medium.com/how-to-hack-your-brain-with-sound-166371c85a66

Smith, J., & Chenoweth, H. (2020, March 3). *Inside the life-changing benefits of sound therapy.* Prevention. https://www.prevention.com/health/mental-health/a30986834/what-is-sound-therapy/

Smith, L. (2019, September 30). *Binaural beats therapy: Benefits and how they work.* Medical News Today. https://www.medicalnewstoday.com/articles/320019#benefits

Solfeggio frequencies - nature healing society. (2019, August 28). Nature Healing Society. https://www.naturehealingsociety.com/articles/solfeggio/

Sound baths are amazing for relaxation so here's how to create your own at home. (2020, November 25). Glamour. https://www.glamour.co.za/wellness/sound-baths-are-amazing-for-relaxation-so-heres-how-to-create-your-own-at-home-911deff4-e799-43a7-bda2-1df6b6d58600

Sound energy: What it is and why it matters to you? (2021, August 30). Amigo Energy. https://amigoenergy.com/blog/sound-energy-what-it-is-why-it-matters/

Sound healing. (n.d.). The Self Love Lab. Retrieved October 25, 2022, from https://theselflovelab.co.uk/pages/sound-healing

Sound healing - sound detox | detox for insomnia | sound meditation. (n.d.). Dhyaana Wellbeing. Retrieved October 19, 2022, from https://dhyaanawellbeing.com/sound-healing/

Sound healing for chakras - yoga signs. (2020, September 3). Yoga Signs. https://yogasigns.com/sound-healing-for-chakras/

Sound healing therapy: What is it and how can it benefit you? (2022, April 12). Sensory Retreats. https://sensoryretreats.com/blogs/news/sound-healing-therapy#:~:text=Music%20or%20sound%20healing%20therapy

Sound healing: Benefits and techniques | miracle-ear. (2021, May 25). Miracle Ear. https://www.miracle-ear.com/blog-news/what-is-sound-healing

Sound masking for healthcare facilities. (2016, December 12). Cambridge - Industry Leading Sound Masking from Biamp. https://cambridgesound.com/healthcare/

Sound masking system for offices & healthcare facilities. (2022, March 14). Soft DB. https://www.softdb.com/sound-masking/

Sound therapy for addiction treatment and rehabilitation. (2016, December 12). Windwardway. https://windwardway.com/addiction-treatment-program/sound-therapy/

Sparrow, J. (2021, September 1). *Sound frequency the power to healing your mind, body and soul.* Sheen Magazine. http://www.sheenmagazine.com/sound-frequency-the-power-to-healing-your-mind-body-and-soul/

Spectral Binaural Beats Meditation. (2018). Get rid of all skin problems | rife frequency for acne, allergy, pimples, eczema, all skin disease [YouTube]. In *YouTube.* https://www.youtube.com/watch?v=m2GOZ7HYWPA

Spicer, S. (2018, June 6). *How binaural beats can heal your mind & body?* LinkedIn. https://www.linkedin.com/pulse/how-binaural-beats-can-heal-your-mind-body-dr-susan-susie-spicer/

Summer, J. (2018, October 29). *White noise: How how to use it for better sleep.* Sleep Foundation. https://www.sleepfoundation.org/noise-and-sleep/white-noise

Sutevski, D. (2020, September 23). *Sound marketing: Using audio branding to strengthen your small business.* Entrepreneurship in a Box. https://www.entrepreneurshipinabox.com/22553/sound-marketing-using-audio-branding-strengthen-small-business/

Suttie, J. (2017). *How music helps us be more creative.* Greater Good. https://greatergood.berkeley.edu/article/item/how_music_helps_us_be_more_creative

Tamsyn. (2012, October 2). *Movable "do" vs fixed "do."* Teaching Children Music. https://www.teaching-children-music.com/2012/10/movable-do-vs-fixed-do/

Tellinger, M., & Heine, J. (2009). *Temples of the african gods : Decoding the ancient ruins of southern africa.* Zulu Planet Publishers. https://unitedvibrations.wordpress.com/michael-tellinger/ (Original work published 2008)

The basics of soundscaping. (2021, June 22). Acoufelt. https://acoufelt.com/sound-advice/soundscaping/

The best sound healing instruments for beginners - SHA blog. (2022, August 17). Sound Healing Academy. https://www.academyofsoundhealing.com/blog/a-guide-to-the-best-sound-healing-instruments-for-beginners

The healing power of your voice - holistic voice therapy - BAST. (2015, March 26). The British Academy of Sound Therapy. https://www.britishacademyof soundtherapy.com/the-healing-power-of-your-voice/

The history of sound waves. (2014, February 23). The Music around Us. https:// musicalsoundwaves.wordpress.com/the-history-of-sound-waves/

The human hearing frequency range and audible sounds. (2021, May 10). Nuheara. https://www.nuheara.com/news/human-hearing-frequency-range/

The human hearing range. (2021, June 30). Amplifon; Amplifon. https://www. amplifon.com/au/blog/human-hearing-range

The human hearing range - from birdsong to loud sounds. (2016, October 8). Widex. https://www.widex.com/en/blog/global/human-hearing-range-what-can-you-hear/

The importance of music in different religions - sound infusion. (2020, September 1). Sound Infusion by Cultural Infusion. https://soundinfusion.com.au/ the-importance-of-music-in-different-religions/

The importance of sound effects. (2020, February 20). TopLine Film. https:// toplinefilm.com/blog/the-importance-of-sound-effects

The power of words - compassion international. (n.d.). Compassion. Retrieved October 5, 2022, from https://www.compassion.com/letter-writing/the-power-of-words.htm

The science of brainwaves - the language of the brain. (2019). NeuroHealth Associates. https://nhahealth.com/brainwaves-the-language/

The Uncommon Coach. (2021, August 21). *There is an effective, scientifically backed mental, physical and emotional healing method.* Facebook. https:// www.facebook.com/theuncommoncoach/posts/ pfbid02CXgaYw9SdcNbL3KpYDPxfWtzp9EUsnDBzt4s R6JWTKAFjw996HfpyMYb6piy6rmLl

The use of harmonies in therapeutic sound healing. (n.d.). Sunreed Instrument. Retrieved October 18, 2022, from https://sunreed.com/the-use-of-harmonies-in-therapeutic-sound-healing/

Thompson, D., & WebMD Editorial Contributors. (2016, September 16). *Sound waves: Rx for high blood pressure, migraine?* WebMD. https://www. webmd.com/hypertension-high-blood-pressure/news/20160916/sound-waves-an-rx-for-high-blood-pressure-migraine

Tomasberg, K. (2020, May 3). *Healing sounds of nature.* Guiding Vitality. https://www.guidingvitality.com/blog/healing-sounds-of-nature

TomuTomu. (2015, April 22). *Plant sounds.* YouTube. https://www.youtube. com/watch?v=VvWPT4VhKTk&list= PLCChSdWueYO_vcyunaC1Wc3NBu4ixTjDT

Treasure, J. (2020, August 3). *The 4 ways sound affects us - Julian Treasure.* Julian Treasure. https://www.juliantreasure.com/blog/4-ways-sound-affects

Truini, J. (2019, October 25). *How to soundproof a room.* Popular Mechanics. https://www.popularmechanics.com/home/interior-projects/how-to/ g2470/soundproofing-a-room/

Tuning fork therapy | all body care. (2015, March 31). All Body Care. https:// www.allbodycare.com/tuning-fork-therapy-sound-healing/

Tuning forks – sound healing shop. (n.d.). Sound Healing Shop. Retrieved October 18, 2022, from https://soundhealingshop.com/tuning-forks/

Tyrrell, T. Y. (2019). *Listening with the trees: The subterranean bioacoustics of old growth forest groves in the hoh river valley.* Schumacher College. http:// npshistory.com/publications/olym/tyrrell-2019.pdf

University of Exeter. (2018, May 15). *Evidence shows ocean sound may help reduce stress and create a sense of calm.* Phys. https://phys.org/news/2018-05-evidence-ocean-stress-calm.html

University of Michigan. (2022, April 18). *Tumors partially destroyed with sound don't come back.* ScienceDaily. https://www.sciencedaily.com/releases/ 2022/04/220418093955.htm

Using music to tune the heart - harvard health. (2019, August 26). Harvard Health; Harvard Health. https://www.health.harvard.edu/newsletter_arti cle/using-music-to-tune-the-heart

Van Ness, N. (2020, June 26). *Why sound masking matters in healthcare facilities.* LinkedIn. https://www.linkedin.com/pulse/why-sound-masking-matters-healthcare-facilities-nathan-van-ness/

Vaughan, A. (2019, December 5). *Recordings reveal that plants make ultrasonic squeals when stressed.* New Scientist. https://www.newscientist.com/arti cle/2226093-recordings-reveal-that-plants-make-ultrasonic-squeals-when-stressed/

Verma, S. (2017, September 8). *The healing power of mantras.* Sonima. https:// www.sonima.com/meditation/mindful-living/mantra/#:%7E:text=If% 20you%20have%20repeated%20the

Violy. (2019, November 26). *A comparison of movable do & fixed do.* Medium. https://qinhelper.medium.com/a-comparison-of-movable-do-fixed-do-d0333acb0d25

Wallmann, H., & Vanwye, W. (2016). Musculoskeletal disorders and treatment the effects of an audible low frequency acoustic waveform on osteoarthritis: A pilot study. *J Musculoskelet Disord Treat*, 2(3), 21. https://clinmedjour nals.org/articles/jmdt/journal-of-musculoskeletal-disorders-and-treatment-jmdt-2-021.pdf

Wei, M. (2019, July 5). *The healing power of sound as meditation | psychology today south africa*. Psychology Today. https://www.psychologytoday.com/za/blog/urban-survival/201907/the-healing-power-sound-meditation

Weidenfeld, J. (2014, June 18). *Top 10 amazing uses for sound - listverse*. Listverse. https://listverse.com/2012/11/14/top-10-amazing-uses-for-sound/

What are brainwaves? | improve brain health with neurofeedback. (n.d.). Sinha Clinic. Retrieved October 18, 2022, from https://www.sinhaclinic.com/what-are-brainwaves/

What are brainwaves? Types of brain waves | EEG sensor and brain wave – UK. (2019). Brainworks Neurotherapy. https://brainworksneurotherapy.com/what-are-brainwaves

What does sound therapy have to do with breathing? (2020, December 23). Sound Therapy International. https://mysoundtherapy.com/au/2020/12/23/what-does-sound-therapy-have-to-do-with-breathing/

What is ambient noise? - definition from safeopedia. (2018, November 10). Safeopedia. https://www.safeopedia.com/definition/5568/ambient-noise

What is ambient sound and how to use this function? (n.d.). Panasonic. Retrieved November 1, 2022, from https://support-uk.panasonic.eu/app/answers/detail/a_id/7038/~/what-is-ambient-sound-and-how-to-use-this-function%3F

What is cymatics? The art and science of visible sound explained. (n.d.). Journey of Curiosity. Retrieved October 16, 2022, from https://journeyofcuriosity.net/pages/what-is-cymatics-how-to-explained

What is music therapy? | taking charge of your health & wellbeing. (2016). Taking Charge of Your Health & Wellbeing. https://www.takingcharge.csh.umn.edu/common-questions/what-music-therapy

What is shamanic sound healing? (2018, October 4). EntheoNation. https://entheonation.com/blog/shamanic-sound-healing/

What is the best plant music device? (2020, October 1). PlantWave. https://www.plantwave.com/blog/what-is-the-best-plant-music-device

What is the function of the various brainwaves? (1997, December 22). Scientific American. https://www.scientificamerican.com/article/what-is-the-function-of-t-1997-12-22/

Why is sound important and what does it mean to us? Top 5 reasons why we need sound. (2017, April 7). Woof on the Wall. https://www.woofonthewall.co.uk/blogs/the-sound-art-blog/why-is-sound-important-and-what-does-it-mean-to-us-top-5-reasons-why-we-need-sound

Willis, L. (2017, August 7). *The benefits of sound therapy.* Wellwood Health. https://www.wellwoodhealth.com/wellness/soundtherapy/#:~:text=Sound%20Therapy%20is%20effective%20in

Windus, S. (2019, November 18). *The sound of skin care: Sound healing and the spa.* DermaScope. https://www.dermascope.com/wellness/11302-the-sound-of-skin-care-sound-healing-and-the-spa

Wong, C. (2021, July 14). *The benefits of music therapy.* Verywell Mind; Verywellmind. https://www.verywellmind.com/benefits-of-music-therapy-89829

Wynn, P. (2021, September 21). *Binaural beats for migraine: Benefits & how it works.* Verywell Health. https://www.verywellhealth.com/binaural-beats-migraine-5200206

Yale School of the Environment. (2017, June 24). *What do plants sound like? Plants and the audible spectrum.* YouTube. https://www.youtube.com/watch?v=8gPERvgAQTc

Yao, B. (2021, September 14). *Aging healthy through sound therapy and meditation by bernadette yao.* Asian Women for Health. https://www.asianwomenforhealth.org/blog/september-is-healthy-aging-month

Yee-Litzenberg, L. (2017, September 12). *How music (and mold remediation) helped mia get her groove back.* National Eczema Association. https://nationaleczema.org/blog/journey-music-healing/

Yogananda, P. (2019). *Autobiography of A yogi.* Ancient Wisdom Publicatio.

Zeyl, J. (2020, May 5). *Infrasonic hearing in birds review.* Seabird Acoustics. https://seabirdsound.org/2020/05/05/infrasonic-hearing-in-birds-review/

Zola, A. (n.d.). *What is sound wave? - definition from whatis.com.* WhatIs. Retrieved October 5, 2022, from https://www.techtarget.com/whatis/definition/sound-wave

Zoppi, L. (2020, November 4). *Music therapy: Types and benefits for anxiety, depression, and more.* Medical News Today. https://www.medicalnewsto day.com/articles/music-therapy#how-it-works

Zuber, A. (2019, July 17). *Brainwave states and how you can utilize them to transform your life.* Medium. https://medium.com/@AlexandraZuber/brain wave-states-and-how-you-can-utilize-them-to-transform-your-life-604632fc751d

Zuboff, S. (2021, April 30). *How ultrasound therapy helps arthritis pain and related symptoms.* Pro Healthcare Products. https://www.prohealthcareproducts. com/blog/how-ultrasound-therapy-helps-arthritis-pain-and-related-symptoms/

JOURNAL

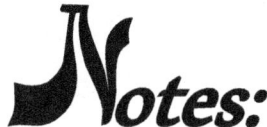

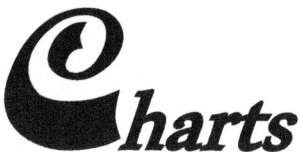

Frequency, Binaural Beat	Immediate Effect	Lingering Effect
		Time: Effect:
		Time: Effect:
		Time: Effect:
		Time: Effect:
		Time: Effect:
		Time: Effect:
		Time: Effect:
		Time: Effect:
		Time: Effect:
		Time: Effect:
		Time: Effect:
		Time: Effect:
		Time: Effect:

Frequency, Binaural Beat	Immediate Effect	Lingering Effect
		Time: Effect:
		Time: Effect:
		Time: Effect:
		Time: Effect:
		Time: Effect:
		Time: Effect:
		Time: Effect:
		Time: Effect:
		Time: Effect:
		Time: Effect:
		Time: Effect:
		Time: Effect:
		Time: Effect:

Frequency, Binaural Beat	Immediate Effect	Lingering Effect
		Time: Effect:
		Time: Effect:
		Time: Effect:
		Time: Effect:
		Time: Effect:
		Time: Effect:
		Time: Effect:
		Time: Effect:
		Time: Effect:
		Time: Effect:
		Time: Effect:
		Time: Effect:
		Time: Effect:

Frequency, Binaural Beat	Immediate Effect	Lingering Effect
		Time: Effect:
		Time: Effect:
		Time: Effect:
		Time: Effect:
		Time: Effect:
		Time: Effect:
		Time: Effect:
		Time: Effect:
		Time: Effect:
		Time: Effect:
		Time: Effect:
		Time: Effect:
		Time: Effect:

Frequency, Binaural Beat	Immediate Effect	Lingering Effect
		Time: Effect:
		Time: Effect:
		Time: Effect:
		Time: Effect:
		Time: Effect:
		Time: Effect:
		Time: Effect:
		Time: Effect:
		Time: Effect:
		Time: Effect:
		Time: Effect:
		Time: Effect:
		Time: Effect:

Frequency, Binaural Beat	Immediate Effect	Lingering Effect
		Time: Effect:
		Time: Effect:
		Time: Effect:
		Time: Effect:
		Time: Effect:
		Time: Effect:
		Time: Effect:
		Time: Effect:
		Time: Effect:
		Time: Effect:
		Time: Effect:
		Time: Effect:
		Time: Effect:

Frequency, Binaural Beat	Immediate Effect	Lingering Effect
		Time: Effect:
		Time: Effect:
		Time: Effect:
		Time: Effect:
		Time: Effect:
		Time: Effect:
		Time: Effect:
		Time: Effect:
		Time: Effect:
		Time: Effect:
		Time: Effect:
		Time: Effect:
		Time: Effect:

Frequency, Binaural Beat	Immediate Effect	Lingering Effect
		Time: Effect:
		Time: Effect:
		Time: Effect:
		Time: Effect:
		Time: Effect:
		Time: Effect:
		Time: Effect:
		Time: Effect:
		Time: Effect:
		Time: Effect:
		Time: Effect:
		Time: Effect:
		Time: Effect:

Playlists

Energizing:

1. _____

2. _____

3. _____

4. _____

5. _____

6. _____

7. _____

8. _____

9. _____

10. _____

11. _____

12. _____

Workout:

1. _____

2. _____

3. _____

4. _____

5. _____

6. _____

7. _____

8. _____

9. _____

10. _____

11. _____

12. _____

Cool Down:

1. _____

2. _____

3. _____

4. _____

5. _____

6. _____

7. _____

8. _____

9. _____

10. _____

11. _____

12. _____

Creativity:

1. _____

2. _____

3. _____

4. _____

5. _____

6. _____

7. _____

8. _____

9. _____

10. _____

11. _____

12. _____

Studying:

1. _____

2. _____

3. _____

4. _____

5. _____

6. _____

7. _____

8. _____

9. _____

10. _____

11. _____

12. _____

Relaxation:

1. _____

2. _____

3. _____

4. _____

5. _____

6. _____

7. _____

8. _____

9. _____

10. _____

11. _____

12. _____

Sleep:

1. _____

2. _____

3. _____

4. _____

5. _____

6. _____

7. _____

8. _____

9. _____

10. _____

11. _____

12. _____

Other: _____

1. _____

2. _____

3. _____

4. _____

5. _____

6. _____

7. _____

8. _____

9. _____

10. _____

11. _____

12. _____

Other: _____

1. _____

2. _____

3. _____

4. _____

5. _____

6. _____

7. _____

8. _____

9. _____

10. _____

11. _____

12. _____

Other: _____

1. _____

2. _____

3. _____

4. _____

5. _____

6. _____

7. _____

8. _____

9. _____

10. _____

11. _____

12. _____

Other: _____

1. _____

2. _____

3. _____

4. _____

5. _____

6. _____

7. _____

8. _____

9. _____

10. _____

11. _____

12. _____

Printed in Great Britain
by Amazon

26497675R00136